Praise for All About Allergies

'Dr Rubin is able to break down th
understandable and actionable steps
this book is also very helpful as a gc
highly recommend *All About Allergies* for anyone wiiu ∪.∪.
dered about their own symptoms.' Kristin Davis, actress and film
producer

'I was a great fan of Dr Rubin's excellent communication style, and
this book really did not disappoint. It has been written with real
clarity by a doctor who clearly knows allergy inside out but who also
has a passion to educate his patients and their families. Engaging
and full of little stories to illustrate his points, this book is perfect
for those who really want to understand their allergy. I think patients will love this as there is a level of detail that will completely
change the way they can talk to their own specialist. I will cer-
tainly be recommending it to my own patients when they tell me
they want to know more.' Professor Adam Fox OBE, Professor of
Paediatric Allergy at Guy's & St Thomas' Hospitals. Trustee & Immediate Past President of British Society for Allergy & Clinical Immunology

'Dr Rubin's book covers a wide variety of allergic conditions, using
a personable, compassionate, and scientific approach enhanced by
storytelling and case examples throughout the text. He cuts through
confusion and misinformation, empowering patients with clear and
trustworthy knowledge to better advocate for their health. This definitive guide is a must-have for the allergy community and promises
to be an invaluable resource for patients and their families.' Professor George Du Toit, Professor of Paediatric Allergy, Evelina Children's London, Guy's and St Thomas' NHS Trust, Kings College
London and a senior author on the LEAP Studies

'In *All About Allergies*, Dr Zachary Rubin delivers the clear, compassionate, and evidence-based guide we've all been waiting for. Whether you're dealing with asthma, food allergies, eczema, or hay fever, this book breaks down the science in a way that empowers you to make informed decisions and advocate for yourself or your family. This is the must-have resource for parents, patients, and anyone who's ever felt lost in the allergy aisle of the pharmacy. If you're ready to take control of your health or support someone you love, start here.' Dr Mary Claire Haver, MD, FACOG, MCP, *New York Times* bestselling author of *The New Menopause*

'With clear, down-to-earth explanations and practical tips, this book demystifies everything from pollen to peanuts—no medical degree required.' #1 *New York Times* bestselling author Abby Jimenez

All About
ALLERGIES

How to Live Well with Asthma,
Food Allergies,
Hay Fever and More

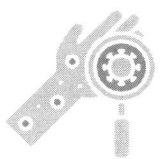

Dr Zachary Rubin

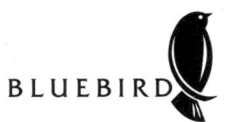

BLUEBIRD

First published 2026 by Plume
an imprint of Penguin Random House LLC

First published in the UK 2026 by Bluebird
an imprint of Pan Macmillan
The Smithson, 6 Briset Street, London EC1M 5NR
EU representative: Macmillan Publishers Ireland Ltd, 1st Floor,
The Liffey Trust Centre, 117–126 Sheriff Street Upper,
Dublin 1 D01 YC43

Associated companies throughout the world

ISBN 978-1-0350-9098-3

1 3 5 7 9 8 6 4 2

A CIP catalogue record for this book is available from the British Library.

Illustrations by Paul Girard

Printed and bound in the UK using 100% Renewable Electricity by CPI Group (UK) Ltd

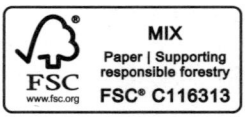

Visit **www.panmacmillan.com/bluebird** to read more about
all our books and to buy them.

*For everyone who has navigated their health with courage,
even when they were misunderstood or unheard—
this book is dedicated to you.*

Contents

PART THREE

Treatment Options

You Are Not Alone

G rowing up, I had a cow's milk allergy, eczema, and seasonal allergies. My cow's milk allergy disappeared early on, but I dealt with eczema throughout my childhood. I could never wear jeans as a kid because the fabric irritated my skin so much, so I had to wear chinos every day. That, combined with thick glasses and a bowl cut, gave me the stereotypical "nerd" look.

Don't get me wrong, being a nerd rules, but in pop culture, a nerd has been synonymous with being weak, a loser, and clutching an inhaler. Think of Milhouse from *The Simpsons*, Mikey from *The Goonies*, and Stevie from *Malcolm in the Middle*. In *Hitch*, Albert either clutches his inhaler or uses it whenever he sees his crush, Allegra. However, when he throws his inhaler away, he finally has the courage to kiss her. It appears that his asthma is "in his head" and he can get what he wants only when he overcomes his anxiety. Like most allergic diseases, asthma is complicated and highly misunderstood, yet these diseases affect millions of people. People who do not live with these diseases may not realize how severe or life-threatening they can be for someone.

Today, despite being a nerd who spent high school more focused on learning to play the trumpet and hula hooping than impressing my classmates, I am a double board-certified pediatrician specializing in allergy treatment and immunology, who reaches millions on social media, where I raise awareness about allergic diseases and how they can be treated. My food allergies and eczema have resolved, but I still have some lingering symptoms of seasonal allergies that are under much better control, especially around dogs and cats. I never thought that I could have three dogs, but I have used what I have learned over the years to manage my allergies well.

I fell in love with medicine early on because I grew up being immersed in the field. I was fortunate because my dad is a pediatrician, so I spent a lot of time in his clinic and observing the impact that he had on his patients and their families. He was solving complex problems, helping families, and getting to know them along the way.

I wanted to be like my dad.

He told me many stories about when he was a medical student. His first lesson in medical school was about chest X-rays. His professor talked about a patient who died because he choked on a fishbone that, because it was made of cartilage, was difficult to identify on a chest X-ray. He talked a lot about the pace and expectations of medical school, and we realized that because technology had changed so much, medical education had likely changed a lot from when he was a student.

There were no premedical courses or clubs at my high school, so we decided to put in a lot of research to develop our own course, called Dr. Rubin's Mini Medical School. My dad tested the curriculum on me to see if I could understand it as a high school student, and I became his first teaching assistant. The program was an eighteen-hour course separated into six sessions that had lectures and hands-on activities. I learned various physical examination and basic procedural skills that I helped teach to my classmates. I not only felt that medicine was my calling, but I also needed to find some capacity to teach.

Fast-forward to my third year in medical school; I tried keeping an open mind about what specialty I would pursue in residency. I thought about gastroenterology, dermatology, and radiology. Ultimately, I picked general pediatrics. While my experiences with my dad influenced me, pediatrics appeared to be a good fit with my personality and how I wanted to help people, especially children.

In my fourth year of medical school, plans quickly changed. I did an elective rotation in allergy/immunology, and I immediately fell in love with the specialty. Outside of a series of lectures on basic immunology, medical school did not dive into the breadth and depth of allergy. The diseases were complex, and the treatment options were expanding rapidly. I really liked the idea of practicing more preventive medicine and helping keep people out of the hospital as much as possible. It was also a bonus that I would be able to take care of people of all ages, so I could still see my pediatric patients when they were grown up.

After three years of general pediatrics residency, I completed two years of a fellowship in allergy/immunology. However, the beginning of the COVID-19 pandemic occurred right as I was transitioning from my fellowship training to my first job at a private practice. I had moved to a new state and there were limited connections for me. Social events were canceled, and primary care clinics were in survival mode. I decided to start posting on social media to connect with people locally.

At first, I was posting on Twitter (now X) and then I switched to TikTok, Instagram, and YouTube. This helped me connect with people locally. However, I quickly realized that there was a lot of incorrect health information (also known as misinformation) on social media, and I was seeing the effects of this misinformation in my clinic. One time, I met a parent who was putting povidone iodine in their child's nose when their child was sick because they had seen it recommended on social media. Currently, we do not know the risks of putting iodine in a child's nose, and there is no substantial evidence that it can help children.

I decided that I would focus on creating educational content that would either address health misinformation or teach people about a medical topic, such as how to use a nasal spray or epinephrine auto-injector, and why you could be allergic to exercise.

I also helped clarify people's stories posted on social media about their health to provide more clinical information. There seemed to be an endless number of stories to talk about:

- Facial swelling while exercising

- A meat allergy due to a tick bite

- Hives all over after being outside in the cold

- An asthma attack

- Sneezing attacks that would make people giggle

- Allergy to water

- Children suffering from a severe allergic reaction after eating food

- Accidentally injecting an EpiPen into their thumb

- Parents introducing foods to their babies outside an emergency room

- Showing off allergy skin test results

The list kept going and going.

Have any of these scenarios happened to you? After spending a lot of time creating educational content, I realized that many people have felt that their experiences are unique and they are alone. There are only about 7,000 board-certified allergists in the United States, which means there is only roughly one allergist per 48,000 people. People who live in more rural or remote areas may not have any access to an allergist. I have received countless messages from people asking for help to understand their allergies, but it is unfortunately impossible to help that way.

I have been interviewed for TV and print media numerous times, and I have realized that people are constantly searching for health information from sources other than their doctors. There are not many allergists who get called on by the media for their expertise, but I have become one of the go-to resources to comment on breaking news or to teach the public about a specific topic related to allergic diseases.

Social media can be a great place to connect with other people and gather information. I created a lot of educational content over the years to teach people about various allergic diseases, but it is hard to keep the information organized online. I wanted to find a way to organize the education I have provided on social media.

That is why I decided to write this book.

It is not meant to be a textbook. This book is designed as a tool to help individuals understand the basics underlying allergies, to arm them with the information they need to live happier, healthier lives. The first part of the book sets the stage for understanding allergic diseases by covering the immune system and basic anatomy of allergies. The second part of the book covers in-depth information on most of the allergic diseases, with some myth-busting along the way. The third part of the book goes into more detail about various treatments and what the future may look like. You may choose to read parts of the book that apply to you, or you may choose to read the entire book to gain a better understanding of allergies and your immune system.

A quick medical disclaimer: This book is not meant to be specific medical advice and cannot diagnose your condition. The information in the book is meant to help you better understand your health and how to navigate the healthcare system. Any concerns about your health should be discussed with your doctor. Also, most of the treatments that I discuss are approved by the American Food and Drug Administration (FDA) to ensure that treatments with the highest safety standards and effectiveness are the primary focus. The stories that I share in the book will have the names of the patients changed and minor details altered to help preserve anonymity except in cases involving public figures or stories told in the news.

I cannot tell you how many times I have been told that people have felt "written off" by their doctors because they could not explain what has happened to them. This does not necessarily mean your doctors don't care about you. In medical school, there is very little training on how to diagnose and manage allergic diseases. Sometimes, it can be difficult to find the underlying cause of an ailment. Our understanding of how our immune system abnormally responds to foreign substances is constantly evolving. This book can also help healthcare professionals have a better understanding of allergic diseases.

Millions of people suffer from various allergic diseases. You are not alone. I hope the information contained in this book will help empower you to learn more about yourself and embark on a journey toward better health.

Part One

The Background

 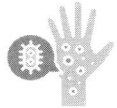

CHAPTER 1

The History of Allergies

Quod ali cibus est, aliis fuat acre venenum.
[What is normal food to one, can be deadly poison for others.]
— **Titus Lucretius Carus (circa 98–55 BC), De Rerum Natura**

When I helped my dad start Dr. Rubin's Mini Medical School, geared toward high school students, he and I created a curriculum that started with the history of medicine. My dad felt that even though many medical schools do not routinely teach the history of medicine, it is crucial to understand where medicine came from so that we have a better understanding of where we go from here. When I was growing up, when my family went on trips outside Illinois, he would take us to medical history museums if they were nearby. I became fascinated with how medicine has evolved so quickly. For example, the first recorded vaccine was given on May 14, 1796, by Edward Jenner to James Phipps, an eight-year-old boy, to protect against smallpox. That was less than 250 years ago!

Allergic diseases are nothing new—they have been around for thousands of years. However, over the past several decades, there has been a dramatic increase in the number of people suffering from these diseases. It is not clear why this is happening. While many people believe these diseases did not exist in the past, there is ample evidence that people have suffered from several conditions, such as food allergies and asthma, since antiquity.

Throughout history, allergies have puzzled and afflicted humanity, shaping our daily lives in ways that are often overlooked. This chapter will focus on the evolution of our understanding of allergies throughout time across the globe. Important historical figures in the field of allergy and immunology will be covered as well. I hope this chapter will spark a curiosity in you that will excite you to learn more about allergic diseases.

Allergies During Ancient Times

The earliest writings in human history are found in ancient Mesopotamia, the area between the rivers Euphrates and Tigris, which is in modern-day Iraq. The Mesopotamians developed a writing system called cuneiform around 3200 BC. They had writings about breathing: *When the patient suffers from cough, he should drink a mixture of Lolium and rose powder dissolved in oil and honey. Afterwards he should eat a broth of pork meat. When he has to defecate, a fire should be lighted where he should direct his anus. Then he will be cured.*

Some of the earliest physicians documented in human history came from ancient Egypt. The first is usually considered to be Imhotep during the 3rd dynasty at around 2600 BC. Two hundred years later, Ni-Ankh-Sekhmet was a physician to King Sahura during the 5th dynasty and is considered to be the first documented allergist. There is a stone at the tomb of the Pharaoh with the inscription "he cured the noses of the kings." One of the oldest Egyptian medical texts, the Papyrus Ebers, was written around 1550 BC and contains twenty-one prescriptions for cough or difficulty breathing (i.e., dyspnea). Some of the ingredients listed include honey, dates, incense, juniper, and beer. A lot of the treatments described may have been used to treat asthma. Honey has been proven to help relieve a cough, but most of these remedies were ineffective for asthma treatment.

Ancient Chinese medicine used various plants to treat airway diseases, including wolfsbane and jimsonweed. A text titled *Su Wen* (meaning "Open Questions") discussed through dialogue between the Yellow Emperor Huangdi and his minister Qi Po a disease that may have been asthma. One passage described how it was helpful to "avoid eating and drinking cold things and one should not wear chilly clothing." We know today that one of the most common triggers for asthma symptoms is cold temperatures. One of the earliest descriptions of food allergy came from China. In the text *Shi Jin-Jing* (meaning "Interdictions Concerning Food"), the Chinese emperors Shen Nong and Huangdi advised pregnant women to avoid foods such as shrimp and meat. Individuals with certain skin lesions that may have been eczema were also advised to avoid certain foods. One of the earliest descriptions of urticaria, also known as hives, is more than two thousand years old and comes from China, where it was referred to as Feng Yin Zheng (wind-type concealed rash), which is similar to one of today's traditional Chinese medical terms, Feng Sao Yin Zhen (wind itch concealed rash). Wind in traditional Chinese medicine is considered to be a major factor for developing urticaria, so other names for urticaria are Feng Zhen Kuai (wind rash lumps) and Feng Zhen (wind rash).

The father of medicine is generally considered to be the Greek physician and philosopher Hippocrates (circa 460–377 BC). In a collection of over sixty of his medical works, called the *Corpus Hippocraticum*, there is no mention of allergic rhinitis. While it is possible that it did not exist in ancient Greece, the more likely explanation is that the symptoms were not severe enough to warrant the attention of physicians. Asthma was described in this text ten times, and there is one passage that refers to the breathing noise as "if somebody was whistling through a pipe." Hippocrates also described how you could be allergic to exercise: "After exercise the pain occurs in one or another area on the chest or the back and the body will be covered with wheals like after contact with nettles." This passage also infers the concept of contact urticaria. Hippocrates used the word *knidosis* to describe urticaria. He also observed that some people reacted strangely after eating cheese, which likely referred to a food allergy.

There were some famous individuals who may have suffered from allergic diseases in antiquity. The first likely documented case of a fatal allergic reaction known as anaphylaxis has been attributed to Pharaoh Menes in 2641 BC. Hieroglyphs from his tomb indicate that he probably died after a sting from a wasp, a cause of death that in most cases is due to anaphylaxis. Roman Emperor Augustus likely suffered from asthma, allergic rhinitis, and eczema. His great-nephew, Emperor Claudius, suffered from allergic rhinitis. Britannicus, the son of Claudius, apparently suffered from an allergy to horses.

Allergies in the Middle Ages and Renaissance

Significant medical advancements came from the Middle East during the Middle Ages. Abu Bakr al-Razi (865–932), also known as Rhazes, was a Persian physician who gave the first description of "rose fever" in his paper "Dissertation regarding the course of Coryza occurring in spring when the roses emit their odor." The descriptions of rose fever are similar to the symptoms of allergic rhinoconjunctivitis. This concept became pervasive during the Middle Ages. German physician Veit Riedlin (1656–1724) performed provocation tests: He hid a pouch of rose leaves in the coat of his patient without their knowing, to see if symptoms were reproducible.

The Jewish physician Moses Maimonides (1135–1204) was the personal physician to Sultan Saladin in Egypt. He wrote a thesis on treating asthma, and many of his recommendations are relevant even today. Maimonides recommended personal hygiene, relaxation, exercise, massage, and avoiding noxious environmental triggers and drugs such as opium. He also recommended that patients with asthma avoid foods such as milk, nuts, and chicken.

Food allergies may have influenced a famous figure in English history. Sir Thomas More (1478–1535), who was a lawyer, reported that King Richard III of England (1452–1485) was sensitive to straw-berries because they would cause him to experience hives. The king used this reaction in front of his council to claim that his political opponent Lord William Hastings was trying to poison him, so he had Hastings executed.

Up until the nineteenth century, skin disorders were not considered to be a problem, because it was believed that the skin was an organ meant to eliminate waste from the body. Therefore, skin eruptions—especially oozing ones—were considered to be beneficial. Physicians for most of human history did not want to treat skin diseases, because they thought it was dangerous to try to heal them. This belief was based on the humoral theory, which has often been credited to Hippocrates, though the theory predates him. In his theory, the human body contains four humors: blood, phlegm, yellow bile, and black bile. If these humors are out of balance, then diseases will occur. This theory was replaced by germ theory by the end of the nineteenth century.

Allergy During the Nineteenth Century

Major strides in our foundational understanding of allergy and immunology started in the nineteenth century. The first thorough description of allergic rhinitis came from John Bostock (1773–1846), who initially called it catarrhus aestivus in 1819. However, by 1828, the more popular term, *hay fever*, was wide spread and is still used today. At that time, it was believed that the smell of hay during the summer and harvest months caused the symptoms. In the 1870s, Charles Blackley (1820–1900) identified the cause of hay fever to be pollen. He invented devices to measure pollen in the atmosphere as well as the first skin-testing devices.

While asthma had been described in the medical literature numerous times at this point, the first classical descriptions of asthma came in 1860 from English physician Henry Hyde Salter (1823–1871). His explanation of asthma was based on hundreds of cases he had seen and his personal experience with the disease. Salter's definition of asthma was "paroxysmal dyspnoea of a peculiar character, generally periodic with intervals of healthy respiration between the attacks." He believed that asthma was a nervous disorder, a notion that has been perpetuated in popular culture even to this day. However, Salter also knew that asthma was due to many other triggers, such as exposure to cats and horses. He recommended coffee, which was one of the earliest effective treatments for asthma because caffeine can temporarily relax the muscles in your airways to improve lung function. French physician René Laënnec (1781–1826) invented the stethoscope, which paved the way for the physical diagnosis of chest diseases, including asthma.

Paul Ehrlich (1854–1915) was a Nobel Prize-winning German physician and scientist who was considered one of the fathers of immunology, specifically of the humoral adaptive immune system. His work in staining cells under a microscope led to his discovery of the mast cell in 1878, which is an important cell in causing allergic reactions. Ehrlich initially named them *Mästzellen*; he thought these cells had a nutritional function because of the granules inside them. The German word *maesten* means to stuff or force-feed. A year later, Ehrlich discovered eosinophils, which are white blood cells that are also important in causing allergic reactions. He was the first scientist to develop a medication to treat syphilis; it was an arsenic-based compound called Salvarsan. To top it all off, Ehrlich coined the term *chemotherapy*.

The Russian immunologist Elie Metchnikoff (1845–1916) won the Nobel Prize for his work in immunology. He is considered the father of cell-mediated immunity. This is the arm of the immune system involving immune cells that do not use antibodies. In 1883, he published his first paper on our understanding of phagocytosis, which is the process in which cells ingest foreign substances and other cells. He noticed that foreign materials were being engulfed by the cells of a transparent starfish larva. These cells were called phagocytes, a term derived from the Greek *phagein*, meaning "to eat," and *cyte*, meaning "cell." Metchnikoff also coined the term *gerontology* and is widely recognized as a pioneer in the study of aging. He even theorized that probiotics could improve health and delay aging.

Allergy at the Start of the Twentieth Century

The major breakthroughs in the field of allergy came at the beginning of the twentieth century. In 1902, Charles Richet (1850–1935) and Paul Portier (1866–1962) used a lab on the yacht *Princesse Alice II*, which belonged to the prince of Monaco, Albert I, to study *Physalia* (Portuguese man of war). If you are not familiar with these animals, they are hydrozoans that look like jellyfish. One of their extracts contains a substance called hypnotoxin, which causes painful hives when skin comes into contact with it. Sailors were accustomed to these uncomfortable stings. While on the voyage, Richet and Portier tried to immunize dogs against this toxin by administering small doses on multiple occasions. However, the opposite occurred. One dog in the experiment, named Neptune, had received two doses of the toxin three days apart that were well tolerated. After twenty-two days, he received the same dose for a third time, but within seconds after the injection, Neptune began to gasp and wheeze, vomited blood, and passed away within twenty-five minutes. Richet initially called this phenomenon aphylaxis because of the "lack of protection" from this reaction, but the name was quickly changed to anaphylaxis because it was more appealing. *Anaphylaxis* is the term describing a severe, potentially life-threatening allergic reaction. Richet ended up winning the Nobel Prize in 1913 for this discovery.

The word *allergy* was coined in 1906 by Clemens von Pirquet (1874–1929), an Austrian pediatrician. He wrote in the journal *Münchener Medizinische Wochenschrift* that "we need a new . . . word for the altered state which the organism finds out by the acquaintance with any organic, living or lifeless poison . . . For this general concept of altered responsiveness, I suggest the term allergy." The older term, *idiosyncrasy*, was replaced very quickly from this point by *allergy*, from the Greek word *allos* (other) and *ergos* (activity). Pirquet also coined the term *allergen* to describe substances that—upon repeated exposure—lead to a reaction. His initial observations came around 1902 when he took care of children who developed side effects when given horse serum antitoxin to treat diphtheria. He was also a pioneer in medical education. He placed a high value on teamwork between doctors and patients and insisted that his trainees finish a nursing training period to understand problems and take care of patients better.

The word *atopy* was coined by Arthur Fernandez Coca (1875–1959) and Robert Anderson Cooke (1880–1960) in the 1920s. This concept describes how there is a genetic tendency to develop allergic diseases such as asthma, eczema, and allergic rhinitis. Sometimes, *atopy* refers generally to any allergic reaction caused by the antibody called immunoglobulin E (IgE).

Finding the Source of Allergic Reactions

Throughout the early twentieth century, many steps were taken to try and find the source of reactions that were observed. This substance was often referred to as the reagin. In 1919, a thirty-five-year-old waiter with no significant medical history developed anemia and received a blood transfusion. Two weeks later, he entered a horse carriage at Central Park in New York City and developed an asthma attack five minutes later. He was given epinephrine and his symptoms resolved. However, the next day he entered the park and developed a similar asthma attack. He was then seen by Dr. Maximilian Ramirez, who did a battery of allergy tests and found that the young man was allergic to horses. It turned out that the blood donor for this patient was an asthmatic who was also allergic to horses. This showed that the allergy had been transferred to the patient by the blood donation.

The transfer of allergies is a phenomenon that still exists today. I once saw an elderly patient named Gerald, who had a history of leukemia that had required a stem cell transplant several years prior to seeing me. The good news was that his cancer went into remission. The bad news was that the donor had a history of allergies to milk and eggs. Gerald developed a condition called transplant-acquired food allergies. He came to me to determine whether his food allergies had been resolved. Unfortunately, the testing determined that he was still allergic to these foods. While this phenomenon is not common, it is important for people to be aware that this can potentially happen.

In 1922, Carl Prausnitz (1876–1963) and his assistant Heinz Küstner (1897–1963) published that allergies can be transferred using serum, which is the component of blood that does not have cells or play a role in clotting. Küstner was allergic to fish, and Prausnitz was allergic to pollen but not allergic to fish. They decided to draw Küstner's blood and inject his serum into Prausnitz's skin. The next day, fish extract was injected near the injection sites of Küstner's serum and around other areas. Only the areas near Küstner's serum reacted quickly with a hive. Clearly, there was a substance being transferred that led to allergic reactions. This method became known as the Prausnitz-Küstner test, which was the classic method for quantifying specific allergen antibodies for many decades.

Not until 1967 did two independent groups of researchers discover the source of many of these allergic reactions, which was IgE. The *E* in *immunoglobulin E* refers to the antibody's ability to create erythema, which is a red skin condition. Kimishige Ishizaka (1925–2018) and Teruko Ishizaka (1926–2019) isolated IgE from people allergic to ragweed pollen. At the same time, S. G. O. Johansson and H. Bennich identified an unknown antibody in a patient with myeloma, which they named after the patient's initials, IgND. The IgE and IgND antibodies were the same substance. The World Health Organization decided to keep the name IgE, which is still used today.

Allergy Testing

Prior to the work by Charles Harrison Blackley in the 1870s, there were hardly any experiments or testing available for studying allergies. Blackley developed the scratch test on the skin in 1873, when he tested timothy grass on his own skin and first described the test. In 1882, German scientist Robert Koch (1843–1910) uncovered the bacteria that cause tuberculosis. By 1890, he discovered tuberculin, which is a substance derived from the tuberculosis bacterium that could be used for skin testing. Pirquet modified the tuberculin test by placing a drop of tuberculin on the skin of the forearm and then using his "Pirquet drill" to scratch that area of skin. This was the precursor to the skin prick test devices that are used today.

The first skin test used to diagnose a food allergy was performed by American pediatrician Oscar Menderson Schloss (1882–1952). He used a scratch test with hen's egg white to prove that a patient was allergic to eggs. Schloss also was able to test for oatmeal and almond allergies. The discovery of IgE paved the way for blood testing for food allergies. Oral food challenges, which are considered the gold standard for diagnosing food allergies through careful observation of reactions to eating a potential food allergen, have been performed at least since 1926. At that time, a fatal reaction tragically occurred in an eighteen-month-old with eczema who had had three episodes previously of an allergic reaction after eating pease pudding. This is an English dish that mainly consists of boiled yellow split peas, water, salt, and spices. The toddler was given a carrot/pea mixture by the head nurse at a pediatric hospital during their lunch break to determine whether he would react. Immediately, the child developed swelling, had difficulty breathing, and died.

The "modified prick test," which is used today, was developed by Helmtraut Ebruster (1922–1996) in Austria. This test was published in 1959 and has become one of the most used allergy tests globally. The procedure involves placing a drop of allergen extract on the skin, usually the forearm or back, and then gently pricking the skin through the drop with a sterile needle or lancet. This completely revolutionized allergy testing at the time. However, despite her tremendous contributions, Ebruster is often referred to as the "forgotten author" of the modified prick test. I spent a tremendous amount of time searching for more information on her, but there was little I could find. She deserves more recognition for her contributions to medicine.

In 1961, Spanish physician Alberto Oehling (1928–2014) developed the "rub test." An allergen was rubbed directly on the skin to observe whether a skin reaction would occur. While this was an easy procedure to perform, it was not necessarily a reliable test because the amount of allergen applied varied significantly. The pressure and duration of rubbing was not standardized, so it was a difficult test to interpret. Many tests resulted in a false negative result because the allergen did not always penetrate the skin deeply enough to elicit a reaction.

The patch test that is used for diagnosing contact dermatitis (see chapter 9) was first introduced by German dermatologist Josef Jadassohn (1863–1936) in 1894. This test places substances on the back that are covered for several days to see if a delayed rash occurs. Around 1928, the patch test was further developed by Bruno Bloch (1878–1933). Initially called the Jadassohn-Bloch patch test, it became known as simply the patch test by 1931.

In 1851, William P. Kirkman (1827–1852), a British physician with a history of hay fever, sniffed the pollen from a grass in his greenhouse, causing a severe bout of sneezing for the next hour. This was the first recorded case of a nasal provocation test, which involves applying a suspected allergen directly into the nose to see if symptoms are produced. While the nasal provocation test is not widely used today, it is often used in research settings and to confirm workplace-related allergies if other tests are inconclusive.

Allergy Treatments

In 1911, British scientist Sir Henry Dale (1875–1968) discovered histamine, which is the chemical responsible for many symptoms related to allergies (see chapter 2). Pharmacologists Daniel Bovet (1907–1992) and Anne-Marie Staub (1914–2012) worked together to search for a drug that could block the effects of histamine, that is, an antihistamine. They discovered the first substance known to have antihistamine properties, called thymoxyethyldiethylamine. The first antihistamine medication to be used clinically was phenbenzamine, which was introduced by Bernard Halpern (1904–1978) in 1942. This was followed by diphenhydramine in 1945. The first generation of antihistamines came out in the 1940s and 1950s (see chapter 15), but these medications had other effects on the body, including blocking a neurotransmitter called acetylcholine (thus, anticholinergic). These side effects led pharmaceutical companies to search for other drugs. For example, while chlorpromazine (Thorazine) is an antihistamine, it is used to treat psychiatric disorders such as schizophrenia and bipolar disorder. This medication is not traditionally used to treat allergies.

Many side effects were reported with the first-generation antihistamines, such as sedation, so the search for antihistamines that mainly blocked histamine intensified in the 1970s and 1980s. The initial second-generation antihistamines discovered were terfenadine and astemizole. However, these medications are no longer in use because they were found to cause an increased risk of cardiac arrest. The newer second-generation antihistamines such as loratadine (Claritin) and fexofenadine (Allegra, Telfast) were released in the 1990s and are still widely used today.

Glucocorticoids, a type of steroid hormone produced by the adrenal glands, have multiple functions, including anti-inflammatory effects as well as influencing growth and mood. Cortisol is an example of a glucocorticoid. In 1900, a physician from Philadelphia named Solomon Solis-Cohen (1857–1948) reported that adrenal gland extract taken by mouth helped treat asthma. Later, Edward Kendall (1886–1972) won the Nobel Prize in 1950 for isolating several steroids from the adrenal cortex in the 1940s, including cortisone—which was known as "compound E" at the time—and adrenocorticotropic hormone (ACTH). Philip Hench (1896–1965) shared this Nobel Prize with Kendall because he used cortisone and

ACTH to treat patients with rheumatoid arthritis. Using steroids to treat inflammatory diseases became very popular moving forward.

The first placebo-controlled clinical trial in the UK using cortisol to treat asthma was not successful in the 1950s. However, higher doses of oral steroids became popular to use, but significant side effects were reported, including metabolic problems, osteoporosis, and stunted growth in kids. Therefore, scientists became interested in developing inhaled steroids with less potential for severe side effects. Initially, scientists tried cortisone and dexamethasone, but these medications did not work well topically in the lungs. The first effective inhaled steroid to treat asthma, beclomethasone dipropionate, was discovered in the 1970s by chemist Sir David Jack (1924–2011). He also invented several other asthma medications that included the bronchodilators salbutamol and salmeterol as well as the inhaled steroid fluticasone propionate. He was also responsible for inventing sumatriptan, a commonly used migraine medication, and ondansetron, which treats nausea and vomiting.

Allergen immunotherapy (see chapter 16), often in the form of shots or drops, is a treatment that helps address the underlying cause of allergic rhinitis, which is an abnormal immune response to environmental allergens such as pollen and pet dander. In 1911, British physician Leonard Noon (1877–1913) published in *The Lancet* the first record of the effectiveness of subcutaneous immunotherapy (SCIT) for people allergic to grass pollen. He also tried to establish a standardized allergen dosing, which he called the Noon unit, based on weight. When he passed away in 1913, his friend John Freeman (1877–1962) continued his work and published another paper three months after Noon's death, which did not report positive results. There were no other clinical trials for SCIT until almost fifty years later, but those clinical trials and beyond showed significant benefits for administering SCIT to treat allergic rhinitis.

In 1975, César Milstein (1927–2002) and Georges Köhler (1946–1995) developed hybridoma technology. This allows scientists to create highly pure and specific antibodies known as monoclonal antibodies, often referred to as biologics (see chapter 17). This break-through has revolutionized research, clinical diagnostics, and therapeutics. Milstein and Köhler went on to win the Nobel Prize in 1984. The first monoclonal antibody that was approved by the FDA was muromonab-CD3 in 1986 for the prevention of acute organ transplant rejection. Omalizumab (Xolair) became the first mono-clonal antibody to be approved by the FDA in 2003 to treat severe allergic asthma. Since then, we have seen a remarkable rise in the number of treatments for various allergic diseases, which we will discuss throughout this book.

In looking back at the history of allergy, we see a journey from ancient observations of mysterious rashes and labored breathing to the modern science of allergy and immunology. What was once thought of as an imbalance of humors is now understood to be a complex relationship between genetics, environment, and an abnor-mal immune response. We have come a long way in our understand-ing of allergic diseases, but there is much to be learned. As you go through this book, you will gain a better understanding of your im-mune system and the allergic reactions that may occur. By the end of the book, we will look into the future to see where we may be heading.

TAKE-HOME POINTS

- While allergic diseases have not been common until modern history, the earliest records indicate that there have always been allergic diseases.

- Major advancements in the study of allergy started in the nineteenth century.

- The term *allergy* was coined in 1906 by Clemens von Pirquet.

CHAPTER 2

The Immune System

This is one of the most important chapters to read in this book, but it may also be the most difficult chapter to read. There is no way around it, because if you are not familiar with the immune system or have never taken an immunology course, then it may not be possible to understand many parts of this book. You can also come back to this chapter at any time if you need a refresher on these concepts.

Understanding the immune system lays the foundation for learning about allergic diseases, since allergies are an abnormal immune system response to foreign substances. While the immune system is designed to protect the body from harmful pathogens such as bacteria, viruses, and cancer, it can mistakenly identify harmless substances such as pollen, pet dander, and food as significant threats. This may lead to an exaggerated immune response that causes a variety of symptoms—from itching and sneezing to potentially life-threatening reactions known as anaphylaxis. By understanding how the immune system works, you will gain critical insight into how and why these reactions occur. This chapter will help you better understand your body.

The format will feel different compared to most of the book because a considerable amount of this chapter covers definitions of terms that are essential for understating allergy and immunology. Some of the information is repeated throughout the book, which I believe will help you remember these concepts. You will not find stories in this chapter like you will in most of the chapters. Instead, there are more analogies to help you understand the concepts better.

What Is the Purpose of the Immune System?

Immunity is a term that means "protection from infectious diseases." The cells and chemicals that help with achieving immunity are the immune system. An antigen is any molecule or substance that can trigger an immune response. The antigen is recognized as foreign by the immune system. An immune response is when the immune system leads a coordinated attack against a foreign substance.

The immune system is vitally important for protecting the body against pathogens, which are tiny disease-causing organisms such as viruses, bacteria, fungi, or parasites. It also protects against various substances that may be toxic to the body, including smoke, heavy metals such as mercury and lead, industrial chemicals, and mycotoxins from mold. When the body sustains an injury, the immune system plays a critical role in the healing process.

When the immune system is trying to protect the body from infection or injury, a cascade of events occurs called inflammation. As an example, if you cut your finger, catch a cold, or eat a food that contains a toxin, your immune system sends a signal to other cells of the immune system to travel to the area of concern. Think of this situation like someone calling 9-1-1 because a building caught on fire. The response by the immune system is to bring specialized immune cells and chemicals to the site of damage and start repairing the damage or fighting off the infection. This is like firefighters rushing to a burning house to put out a fire. This process of inflammation may cause symptoms such as redness, swelling, heat, pain, and/or stiffness. Swelling helps bring extra blood and nutrients to the area, while heat may kill germs. Pain helps you to remember to rest to improve the healing process.

The immune system is also constantly trying to distinguish between "self" and "non-self" to make sure that it is not attacking itself. However, some people may end up developing abnormal immune responses to their own healthy tissue, which is known as autoimmune disease. The immune system must determine whether a foreign substance is harmful. For example, food is a foreign substance, but how does the system know it is safe for the body and is not a pathogen? There are a series of complicated checks and balances to help make eating food safe for most people. When cells in your body are dividing, they may mutate or change into a nonfunctional cell that grows uncontrollably. These are cancer cells, which the immune system may be able to identify and eradicate prior to causing severe disease.

What Is Cell Signaling?

Cell signaling is how cells in your body communicate with one another. It is a critical part of how your body functions. When cells are talking to one another, they send chemical messengers. These are known as signaling molecules, chemical mediators, or ligands. Cytokines are small proteins involved in the messaging between immune cells; they include interferons, tumor necrosis factor-alpha (TNF-α), and interleukins. As the name implies, interleukins are proteins that signal between white blood cells (WBCs); they are written in shorthand such as IL-4, IL-5, and IL-13. When cell signaling occurs, a ligand is released from a cell to find a receptor that is located either on the same cell or on another cell. A receptor is a protein that is found either on the outside of the cell, called a cell membrane, or inside the cell in the nucleus or cytoplasm; this receptor protein binds to a ligand to send a signal inside the cell to start a response. The interaction between a ligand and a receptor is like a lock-and-key fit, with the ligand acting like a key and the receptor like a lock. There are many ways a cellular response may occur. Examples include changing gene expression, activating or inhibiting enzymes, cell growth and division, or programmed cell death (apoptosis).

What Is the Innate Immune System?

The immune system is typically divided into the innate immune system and the adaptive immune system. While these branches of the immune system have distinct characteristics and functions, they do overlap and work together. The first line of defense is the innate immune system. It provides an immediate, nonspecific response to pathogens. The innate immune system is present at birth and does not require an earlier exposure to a pathogen to be activated. The components of the innate immune system include physical barriers such as the skin, stomach acid, and mucous membranes. A mucous membrane is a moist tissue that covers the inside of a body cavity such as the nose, mouth, lungs, and digestive tract. The mucus lining of these cavities traps germs to help prevent infections. There are enzymes such as lysozyme in tears, saliva, and mucus that break down bacterial cell walls.

Another reason why the innate immune system can work very quickly to help prevent an infection is that it can recognize the molecular structures that are on most pathogens; these are called pathogen-associated molecular patterns (PAMPs). Think of your innate immune system like the security system trying to protect against theft at a bank. An immune system cell acts like a security guard. The pathogen would be the burglar and the PAMPs would be the ski mask that covers their face. The security guard would quickly spot the burglar wearing a mask as a potential threat and try to subdue the burglar to prevent theft.

White blood cells, also known as leukocytes, are cells of the immune system that help protect against infection. We will go over some of these WBCs that are relevant to this book. For the innate immune system, neutrophils destroy bacteria and fungi by eating them, through the process called phagocytosis. As noted in chapter 1, cells that can cause phagocytosis are known as phagocytes, which also include monocytes, macrophages, and dendritic cells. Macrophages and dendritic cells are examples of antigen-presenting cells (APCs) because they capture antigens and then show them to the adaptive immune system. Eosinophils attack parasites and release various chemical mediators that may lead to allergic reactions and inflammation.

Mast cells are often seen as cells that cause symptoms of allergies. They also play a role in wound healing and protection against parasites. These cells are located throughout the body and are abundant in tissues that interact with the external environment, including the skin, lungs, and gastrointestinal tract. They are also located near blood vessels and nerves. Mast cells hold granules that store various chemicals and are released during a process called degranulation. These cells can be activated for many reasons that will be discussed throughout many chapters of this book. A couple of triggers of mast cell activation worth mentioning now are physical trauma and emotional stress. The chemical that most people are familiar with is histamine, which can cause blood vessel widening (vasodilation), itching, urticaria (hives), angioedema (swelling), and airways becoming smaller due to smooth muscle contraction (bronchoconstriction). In the gastrointestinal tract, histamine stimulates stomach acid production. Histamine functions as a neurotransmitter in the brain, helping to promote wakefulness and cognitive functions as well as to suppress hunger. There are four histamine receptors: H1, H2, H3, and H4. Antihistamine medications that treat allergies target the H1 receptor. Antacid medications such as famotidine (Pepcid, Pepzan) target the H2 receptor.

There are other substances released by mast cells, including heparin and proteases, which promote vasodilation, inflammation, and tissue remodeling. A protease is an enzyme that breaks down proteins and may promote inflammation. An example of a protease is tryptase, which can be used as a blood test as a marker of mast cell activation. Leukotrienes and prostaglandins promote bronchoconstriction, vasodilation, and increased vascular permeability. Various cytokines are released from mast cells, including IL-4, IL-5, and IL-13, to activate other immune cells and propagate inflammation. Basophils have roles similar to mast cells, but there are significantly fewer basophils present.

The complement system is a group of proteins that have multiple functions. These proteins were discovered in the late nineteenth century by Belgian immunologist Jules Bordet (1870–1961), who found that there are components in the blood that "complement" the antibacterial activity of antibodies. There are over thirty complement proteins, and while you do not need to know them, medical students around the world all struggled to learn them! Complement proteins can mark pathogens for phagocytosis through a process called opsonization. They can form the membrane attack complex (MAC), which is like a drill punching holes into a pathogen's membrane to make it leak and die.

Before we move on to the adaptive immune system, I want to touch on immune complexes because complement proteins help remove them. Immune complexes, also known as antigen-antibody complexes, are molecular structures that form when antibodies bind to antigens. Remember, antigens are foreign substances such as viral proteins or bacterial toxins that can start an immune response. Antibodies, which we will discuss more in the next section of this chapter, are proteins that are produced by the immune system that bind to antigens. Immune complexes help prevent pathogens or toxins from infecting cells in a process called neutralization, promote opsonization, and activate the complement system to clear pathogens. When immune complexes are not cleared effectively, they can deposit in tissues such as joints, blood vessels, or kidneys, which leads to inflammation. Another way to think about immune complexes is as airport luggage. The antigens are luggage bags, while the antibodies are the luggage tags, and the immune complexes form when you have labeled luggage. The complement system and phagocytes are the airport crew that pick up the labeled luggage and remove it from the plane. If there are too many labeled bags or too few workers, then the luggage may pile up before reaching baggage claim.

What Is the Adaptive Immune System?

The adaptive immune system is the specialized arm of the immune system that provides targeted, long-lasting defense against specific pathogens. It takes time for the adaptive immune system to recognize pathogens and learn how to react. Think of the differences between the innate immune system and the adaptive immune system like a security system. The innate immune system is like a security guard who is stationed at the front entrance and will stop anyone they think is suspicious. There is not much need for them to adapt, so their routine is the same every day. On the other hand, the adaptive immune system is like a specialized detective who will identify the specific intruder and develop a tailored plan to stop them. Once they have solved the case, they have a detailed file on the intruder (i.e., immune memory) so they can act quickly and effectively if they return.

The main cells of the adaptive immune system are lymphocytes, which are WBCs responsible for producing antibodies, directly killing tumor cells and virus-infected cells, and regulating the overall immune response. The two main types of lymphocytes are B cells and T cells. B cells are produced in the bone marrow (hence the name B cells) and eventually turn into two main cell types: memory B cells and plasma cells. Memory B cells help remember a specific pathogen after an initial infection or vaccination; they lie dormant in the body for many years and rapidly respond if the pathogen returns. Plasma cells produce large amounts of antibodies during an active infection. They can be short-lived during an infection or long-lived to continuously produce antibodies from the bone marrow to maintain long-term immunity. B cells can also act as APCs (antigen-presenting cells) by ingesting pathogens and presenting them to T cells.

Antibodies, also known as immunoglobulins (Ig), are specialized proteins produced by B cells to help identify and neutralize pathogens. They are Y-shaped structures that are highly diverse. In fact, theoretically, the immune system can produce roughly 10^{15} unique antibodies. There are five types of antibodies: IgG, IgA, IgM, IgE, and IgD. IgG is the most abundant antibody and provides long-term immunity after infection or vaccination. A subclass of IgG antibodies, called IgG4, can have anti-inflammatory and tolerance-inducing effects. As an example, your body produces IgG4 antibodies when you eat food to help your immune system tolerate the food. IgA antibodies are mainly found in mucosal areas such as the respiratory and gastrointestinal tracts as well as saliva, tears, and breast milk. IgM antibodies are the first antibodies produced during the initial immune response to an infection. IgE antibodies provide defense against parasites but are also involved in allergic reactions. IgD antibodies play a role in B cell maturation. Think of antibodies like customized tools crafted for a specific job. Each tool, or antibody, is perfect for handling one specific type of task, or antigen.

T cells are produced in the bone marrow and mature in the thymus (hence the name T cells) and have a variety of functions and subtypes. Helper T cells (CD4+ T cells) activate other immune cells to coordinate an immune response. Cytotoxic, or killer T cells (CD8+ T cells), destroy infected or cancerous cells. Regulatory T cells (Tregs) help promote immune tolerance and prevent autoimmune reactions.

Before moving on, I want to pay special attention to a subtype of helper T cells called T-helper type 2 (Th2) cells because they play a pivotal role in the development of allergic reactions. These cells release IL-4 and IL-13, which are cytokines that cause B cells to produce IgE antibodies. IL-13 also causes mucus production and airway hyperresponsiveness in people living with asthma. Th2 cells also release IL-5, which promotes the activation, recruitment, and survival of eosinophils, which are cells that contribute to inflammation.

What Are Allergic Reactions?

Now that you have a better understanding of the immune system when it comes to protecting against infections, we will dive deeper into how the immune system may abnormally respond to foreign substances. These reactions are often referred to as hypersensitivity reactions. The term *allergy* is broad and does not describe the underlying mechanism—or pathophysiology—for the symptoms that may occur. If you understand the underlying immunologic mechanisms, then allergic diseases become less confusing. Modern medicine relies on gaining an understanding of the pathophysiology of disease so that diagnostic tests and management strategies can be effectively developed.

An important concept regarding allergic reactions is that some symptoms may be more localized to the area of the body that was exposed, while other reactions may involve more than one body part, a response also known as a systemic allergic reaction. Allergic reactions can be either localized or systemic, based on multiple factors, including the type of immune response, the location where the mast cells are activated, and where the allergen exposure occurs in the body. For example, an allergic reaction is more likely to become systemic if the exposure occurs from an injection of an allergen into the blood compared to the allergen being placed on the skin.

Robin Coombs and Philip Gell were immunologists who in 1963 proposed a classification system for hypersensitivity reactions that is still used today. There are four types of hypersensitivity reactions. Type I is the one that most people think about that explains many allergic reactions. This hypersensitivity reaction is mediated by specific IgE antibodies that are produced during the sensitization phase. An allergen is a substance, such as pollen, pet dander, and peanuts, that can cause allergic reactions. During sensitization, APCs such as dendritic cells capture the allergen and present it to a naive T helper cell. Those T cells turn into Th2 cells and influence B cells to produce IgE antibodies that can specifically bind to the allergen.

These antibodies then bind to IgE receptors called FcεRI, which are located on the surface of mast cells and basophils. Once this happens, you are considered sensitized to the allergen. If the immune system sees the allergen in the future, then the allergen may bind to the specific IgE antibodies on the mast cells or basophils in a process called cross-linking. This leads to degranulation, which releases various chemical mediators that we mentioned previously. The symptoms of a type I hypersensitivity reaction vary depending on the site and extent of mast cell and basophil activation. Symptoms usually occur within a few minutes to an hour of exposure and may include sneezing, nasal congestion, runny nose (rhinorrhea), wheezing, shortness of breath, urticaria, angioedema, eczema, or the potentially life-threatening systemic reaction, anaphylaxis. More information regarding testing for type I hypersensitivity reactions will be covered in chapter 4 when we discuss skin and blood testing.

Type II hypersensitivity reactions, also known as cytotoxic hypersensitivity, occur when IgG or IgM antibodies target antigens on the surface of cells or proteins that give a structure to the cells called the extracellular matrix. This leads to cell destruction or tissue damage. There are several diseases that are the result of type II hypersensitivity reactions, which are often categorized as autoimmune diseases. Examples include Graves' disease, which is when antibodies stimulate the thyroid-stimulating hormone receptor, causing hyperthyroidism. This disease often presents with weight loss, heat intolerance, and a fast heart rate (tachycardia). Myasthenia gravis occurs when antibodies block acetylcholine receptors, which causes muscle weakness and difficulty swallowing (dysphagia). A blood transfusion reaction can be a type II hypersensitivity reaction when incompatible blood is transfused, leading to a breakdown of donor red blood cells (hemolysis) by recipient antibodies. This can lead to symptoms of fever, chills, cola-colored urine (hemoglobinuria), and low blood pressure (hypotension).

Type III hypersensitivity reactions occur when immune complexes form and deposit in tissues, such as blood vessels, joints, kidneys, and lungs, leading to inflammation and damage. Once these molecular structures are deposited, they can lead to complement activation, which can recruit other immune cells, such as neutrophils. Examples of type III hypersensitivity reactions include systemic lupus erythematosus, which is the result of immune complexes containing antibodies against DNA or other nuclear components that deposit in the skin, joints, and kidneys. Serum sickness is another disease caused by immune complexes that are often formed from repeated exposure to an antigen such as a medication or vaccine. This can cause immune complexes to deposit in blood vessels and joints. Symptoms may include fever, rash, and joint pain.

A type IV hypersensitivity reaction is often referred to as a delayed hypersensitivity reaction. Unlike type I, II, and III hypersensitivities, delayed hypersensitivity reactions are not mediated by antibodies. The reaction usually takes forty-eight to seventy-two hours after exposure to the antigen, and it is mediated by T cells. The classic example of a type IV hypersensitivity reaction is contact dermatitis, which can occur in response to substances such as nickel, poison ivy, and cosmetics. Chapter 9 will discuss this in more detail.

What Is Immune Tolerance?

If you are allergic to a substance such as cat dander, there is a possibility that you can "outgrow" your allergy. This is called immune tolerance, where the immune system stops having an allergic response when it encounters the substance. There are several potential factors that influence whether someone may develop immune tolerance. Proteins that are easily digested, such as cow's milk and eggs, are more likely to develop tolerance compared to stable proteins such as peanuts or shellfish. Environmental allergens typically are lifelong, but some people may outgrow them. Inconsistent exposure or high-dose exposure to the allergen may worsen the problem, but slow, controlled exposure may help (see chapter 16). A family history of eczema, allergic rhinitis, or asthma (also known as atopy) increases the risk of developing persistent allergies. Allergies may fade over time due to an aging immune system.

Some immunological shifts have been observed during immune tolerance. Regulatory B and T cells produce IL-10, which helps suppress pro-inflammatory T helper cells. Over time, IgE levels decrease while IgG4 levels increase. IgG4 helps induce tolerance to an allergen through several mechanisms. For example, this antibody can bind to allergens to prevent them from cross-linking IgE on the surface of mast cells and basophils. IgG4 almost acts like a sponge to soak up allergens to help prevent an allergic reaction.

We still have a lot to learn about how the immune system becomes hypersensitive and how it becomes tolerant. Once these mechanisms are better understood, we can apply more effective diagnostic and management strategies for allergic diseases. Chapter 18 will go over some of the current research that is happening in the field of allergy. I am proud of you for sticking around to the end of this chapter. The next chapter is the last chapter needed to get a better idea of how the body works so that you will get the most out of this book.

TAKE-HOME POINTS

- The immune system is divided into the innate immune system and the adaptive immune system, which work together to help protect your body from pathogens.

- Antibodies are specific proteins that bind to foreign substances to neutralize them or to activate the immune system.

- There are many mechanisms for an allergic reaction, which dictate the diagnostic tests and treatments that can be offered.

CHAPTER 3

The Anatomy
of Allergies

I want to make sure that you have a basic understanding of not only the immune system but also how it interacts with the physical structures of your body. The immune system is everywhere, so allergic reactions may affect multiple organs differently. We will dive into anatomy in this chapter, which will cover your lymph nodes, bone marrow, ears, nasal and sinus cavities, throat, lungs, gastrointestinal tract, and skin. I will discuss some clinical pearls that relate to anatomy, but these topics may not be directly related to allergic diseases. In medical school, I learned normal anatomy and pathophysiology at the same time to have a better understanding of how the human body functions in normal and abnormal conditions. I believe this learning style will help you gain a better understanding of allergic diseases. Some of the information in this chapter is repeated later in the book to help strengthen your knowledge of these concepts. Just as with chapter 2, you can always come back to this chapter at any point, but first it will help set up foundational knowledge to better tackle the rest of this book.

What Are Lymph Nodes?

Lymph nodes play a critical role in how your immune system responds to foreign substances and regulates itself. They are strategically placed throughout your body, connected by lymphatic vessels, so that the immune system can respond quickly. Think of lymph nodes as water treatment plants for your immune system. Lymph fluid flows into lymph nodes from lymphatic vessels, carrying cellular waste, foreign particles, and pathogens such as bacteria and viruses to the lymph node. There, immune cells act as filters, capturing potentially harmful substances that should not be there. If a pathogen is found, then the immune cells undergo a "treatment process" and start an immune response.

T and B cells that live in the lymph nodes become activated when antigens are presented to them, and they start to divide, expanding the size of a lymph node. As part of the immune response, blood vessels called high endothelial venules become more permeable to allow more lymphocytes into the lymph node. This causes lymph nodes to become larger. You may have noticed that your neck has large bumps when you are sick and they may be painful when you touch them. This means that the lymph nodes in your neck are actively trying to fight off an infection. Enlarged lymph nodes are referred to as lymphadenopathy, which is usually not dangerous if it is due to an infection and resolves within a few weeks. However, there are several features of lymphadenopathy that may be dangerous, including lymph nodes larger than 2 cm in diameter, lymph nodes that remain enlarged for more than two weeks, and lymphadenopathy located just above the clavicle bone, which is the S-shaped bone between the shoulder and the sternum. Firm, hard, or fixed lymph nodes are more likely to be cancerous compared to soft, rubbery, or mobile lymph nodes.

The Bone Marrow

The bone marrow is the soft, spongy tissue inside bone where blood cells are created (i.e., hematopoiesis). It is broadly categorized into two types: red marrow and yellow marrow. Red bone marrow is mostly found in flat bones such as the sternum, ribs, and skull as well as the ends of long bones such as the femur and humerus. There is more red marrow in children than in adults. This is the area of bone marrow that produces red blood cells, white blood cells, and platelets. As people age, some red marrow is replaced by yellow marrow, which is found in the hollow center of long bones. This area is mostly made of fat cells and acts as an energy reserve. In some situations, such as anemia when there is an increased demand for blood cell production, the yellow marrow may be converted into red marrow. In chapter 14, we will explore how cells that originate from the bone marrow, the mast cells we described earlier, may be overproduced, which may require a bone marrow biopsy to uncover the underlying disease.

The Ears

Your ears are responsible mainly for hearing and balance. The anatomy of the ear is divided into three parts: the outer ear, middle ear, and inner ear.

The pinna is the visible part of the ear that collects sound waves and directs them into the ear canal, a tubelike structure that extends to the eardrum (i.e., tympanic membrane). The eardrum is where the middle ear begins, and when sound waves hit this membrane, it vibrates and transmits the energy to the three auditory bones that are connected: the malleus, incus, and stapes. The stapes bone fits next to the oval window, which is the opening to the inner ear. When the stapes moves against the oval window, it moves pressure waves into the fluid-filled cochlea of the inner ear. The cochlea is a tube that looks like a snail, containing hair cells that convert

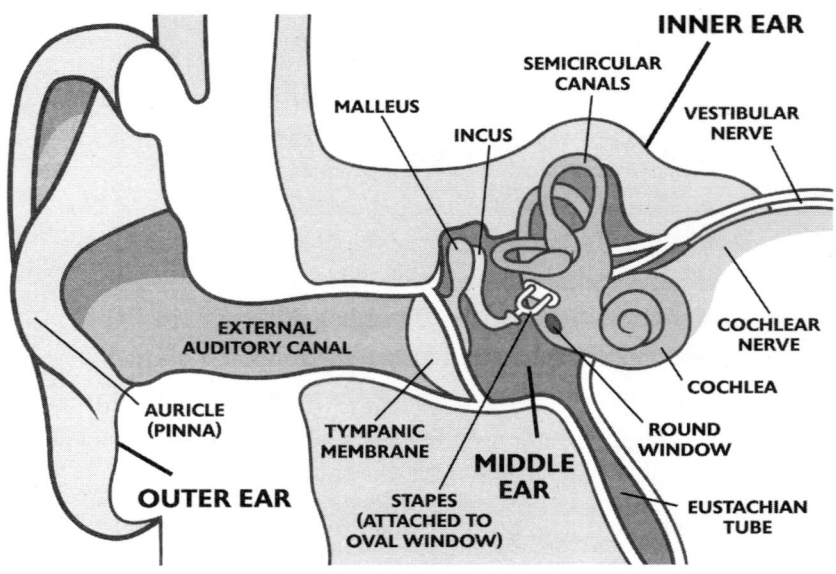

mechanical vibrations from sound waves to electrical signals to the cochlear nerve to the brain, which leads to our perception of sound.

The ear interprets balance through the vestibular system. It contains three fluid-filled loops called semicircular canals that detect rotational head movements. When the head moves, fluid in the semicircular canals moves, stimulating hair cells that send signals to the brain that the head is rotating. The otolith organs include the utricle and saccule, which detect forward motion and head position relative to gravity. The utricle is sensitive to forward and backward movements while the saccule is sensitive to vertical movements such as jumping or falling. Whenever there is movement, calcium carbonate crystals called otoliths move, causing a gelatinous layer underneath the otoliths to shift, which bends hair cells that send signals to the brain that the body is moving.

There is a special structure, the Eustachian tube, that is a narrow passage connecting the middle ear to the upper part of the throat behind the nose. It has several functions. When you are taking an elevator to the top floor of a tall building or flying on an airplane, you may have experienced ear pain. You may have chewed some gum or yawned intentionally to relieve the discomfort. When you do this, you are trying to pop open your Eustachian tubes to equalize the pressure on both sides of your eardrums. The Eustachian tubes help remove mucus, fluids, and debris from the middle ear to prevent fluid buildup. They act like one-way valves to prevent pathogens from the nose and throat from entering the middle ear. However, many children are at risk of developing a middle ear infection (i.e., acute otitis media) because their Eustachian tubes are shorter and oriented more horizontally, so pathogens may travel more easily to the middle ear. Fluid may accumulate in the middle ear after an upper respiratory infection or allergic rhinitis, which is also known as serous otitis media. Treating the underlying cause may help alleviate this issue, but in severe or recurrent cases a set of tubes may be placed in the eardrum to facilitate fluid draining from the middle ear.

The Nose and Sinuses

Your nose has essential roles in sensing smell, facilitating airflow into the lungs, filtering particles and pathogens, humidifying air, and contributing to the quality of your voice. Your external nose contains two openings into the nasal cavity, the nostrils.

While the nose is considered one organ, there are two separate nasal cavities because the nasal septum divides the nasal cavity into left and right nasal passages. In the nasal cavity, bony structures covered with tissue that increase the surface area for air filtration and humidification are called nasal turbinates, which are divided into the inferior, middle, and superior turbinates. Typically, one nostril experiences more airflow than the other due to the nasal cycle, a process in which the nasal cavities alternate between congestion and decongestion. One nasal passage is relatively more obstructed than the other due to the engorgement of erectile tissue. The duration of a nasal cycle ranges usually between one and five hours. If the nasal septum is bent toward one nasal passage (i.e., a deviated nasal septum), then the nasal cycle may worsen the sensation of nasal congestion.

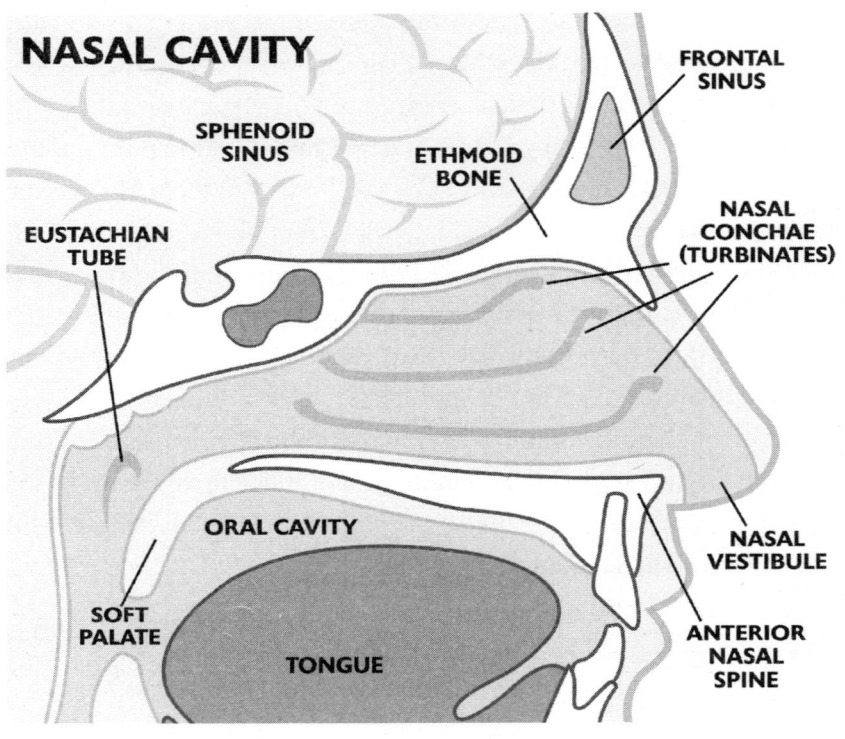

NASAL CAVITY

SPHENOID SINUS

ETHMOID BONE

FRONTAL SINUS

NASAL CONCHAE (TURBINATES)

EUSTACHIAN TUBE

ORAL CAVITY

NASAL VESTIBULE

SOFT PALATE

TONGUE

ANTERIOR NASAL SPINE

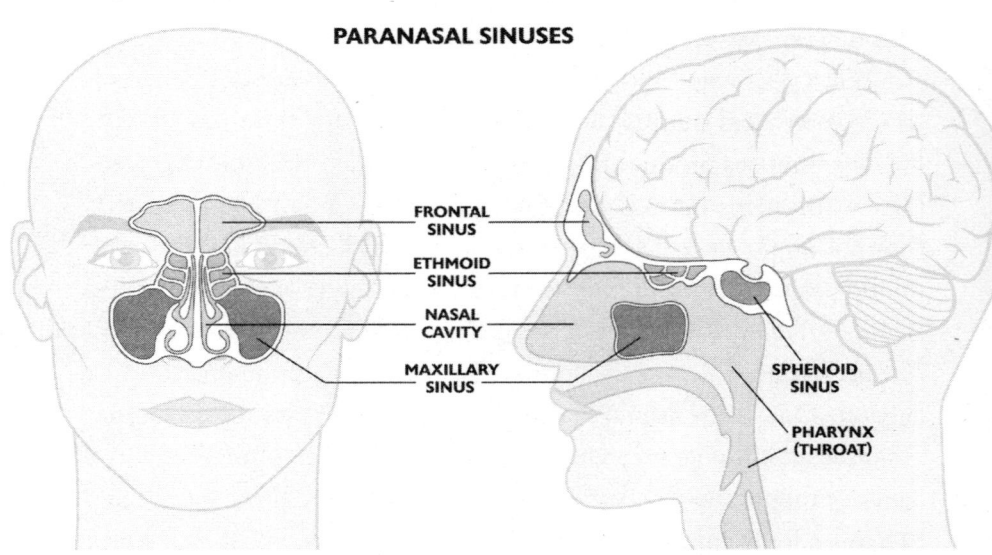

PARANASAL SINUSES

FRONTAL SINUS

ETHMOID SINUS

NASAL CAVITY

MAXILLARY SINUS

SPHENOID SINUS

PHARYNX (THROAT)

The roof of the nasal cavity is where the olfactory nerve is located. This nerve is responsible for sensing smell and may be able to discriminate as many as one trillion unique odors. However, your sense of smell can be lost partially (hyposmia) or completely (anosmia) for several reasons. SARS-CoV-2, the virus that causes COVID-19, can cause anosmia by directly infecting the olfactory nerve. If there is increased inflammation and swelling of the nasal cavity such as for poorly controlled allergic rhinitis or chronic rhinosinusitis, then the olfactory nerve may not be able to sense smell because airflow cannot reach the nerve.

The sinuses are a set of air-filled spaces in the skull that are located around the nose, behind the eyes, cheeks, and forehead. The four sets of sinuses include the maxillary, frontal, sphenoid, and ethmoid sinuses. You are not born with all these sinuses. They do not fully develop until around late adolescence. The maxillary sinuses are the first to develop and are present at birth. The ethmoid sinuses start developing shortly after birth. The sphenoid sinuses start developing at around nine months of age, and the frontal sinuses are the last to start developing, at roughly five to six years of age. These sinuses serve several functions. They help warm, humidify, and filter the air we breathe. These spaces in your skull provide a unique sound to your voice and provide protection to your brain and eyes if there is physical trauma.

The sinuses produce nitric oxide, which has antimicrobial properties and helps improve oxygen uptake. You may have heard that humming may increase nitric oxide levels in the nasal cavity, which could help reduce symptoms of sinusitis and rhinitis. However, there is limited data on whether this works and the only case report that I found reported on one person who had to hum strongly at a low pitch for one hour at bedtime the first night and 60 to 120 times at roughly 18 hums per minute, four times a day for the following four days as treatment for severe chronic rhinosinusitis to see benefit. That is a lot of humming!

Throughout your nose and sinuses, there is mucus, which is

often called snot. Mucus is a slippery, gelatinous fluid that covers mucus membranes, which are found not only in your nose and sinuses but also in other parts of your body, such as your mouth, throat, and gastrointestinal tract. Mucus acts like flypaper and traps foreign particles and pathogens. Hair cells covering the respiratory tract move the debris that is trapped in mucus toward your throat to clean the respiratory tract during a process called mucociliary clearance. An adult typically swallows approximately 1 to 1.5 liters of nasal mucus each day, an amount that can significantly increase during an illness! In addition, nasal mucus contains antimicrobial proteins such as lysozyme and lactoferrin to help fight off pathogens. Mucus also helps prevent tissues from drying out. Mucociliary clearance does not work as well under dry conditions.

Your sinuses also produce mucus to clear pathogens from your respiratory tract. The mucus exits the sinuses through openings called ostia. However, inflammation in the nasal cavity from conditions such as allergic rhinitis or an upper respiratory infection may obstruct the sinus ostia, which disrupts mucociliary clearance. In dry conditions, the hair cells may not work as well, so mucus may accumulate in the sinuses. Upper respiratory infections stimulate more nasal mucus production, which can fill up the sinuses. Excess mucus in the sinuses allows viruses and bacteria to grow, causing an infection known as sinusitis.

The color of your snot may provide clues as to what is going on with your nasal passages. Clear or white mucus is usually seen in people who are healthy or if you have allergic rhinitis. Yellow or green mucus often indicates an infection. These colors occur because neutrophils release enzymes that change the color of the mucus. However, these colors do not reliably distinguish whether the infection is due to a virus or bacteria, so it does not automatically mean you need antibiotics if your snot is green. Red mucus usually means there is blood, which could be from an irritation in your nose, trauma, a foreign body, or potentially a mass in rare instances. Brown or black mucus could be due to a fungal infection or environmental pollutants. We will discuss this topic again in more detail in chapter 6 to frame it in the context of sinusitis.

The Throat

The throat is also known as the pharynx, which is a muscular tube that connects to the respiratory and gastrointestinal tracts. There are three areas of the pharynx. The nasopharynx is the uppermost region of the pharynx, which is above the soft palate in your mouth but near the back of your nose. This is where the Eustachian tube is located. The oropharynx is at the back of your mouth. When you swallow food, the soft palate elevates to close off the nasopharynx to prevent food from moving into your nasal cavity. The laryngopharynx is the lowest point of the throat, where food and air enter the esophagus and larynx, respectively. The epiglottis is the flap of cartilage that covers the larynx when you swallow, to prevent food from entering your lungs.

The tonsils are oval-shaped tissues in the oropharynx, and they are like lymph nodes because they help fight off infections. There are four sets of tonsils: palatine tonsils, pharyngeal tonsils, lingual tonsils, and tubal tonsils. The tonsils that you probably think of when looking at the back of your throat are the palatine tonsils. The pharyngeal tonsils are often referred to as the adenoid, which is in the back of your nasopharynx. When you open your mouth, the soft palate covers the adenoid, so it is not easily visible. Adenoid enlargement is common in children, and it can cause numerous symptoms, including mouth breathing, snoring, frequent ear infections, bad breath, nasal congestion, and sleep disturbances. If left untreated, children may develop a facial developmental abnormality called adenoid facies, which is a long face with an open mouth. Chronic or recurrent infections cause the immune system to be persistently activated, leading to enlargement of adenoid tissue. Allergies may cause chronic inflammation as well. Certain irritants such as tobacco smoke and pollutants can stimulate adenoid enlargement.

The Lungs

Your lungs help exchange oxygen from the air into your blood with carbon dioxide from your blood into the air. This occurs when air is moving into and out of the lungs (i.e., ventilation). Each lung has segments that are known as lobes. The right lung has three lobes while the left lung has two lobes. Think of your lungs as an upside-down tree where there are many branches. The respiratory tract is branched to increase its surface area to maximize gas exchange. When you breathe through your nose or mouth, air travels into the trachea, which is like the trunk of a tree. The two large branches that split off the trunk are called the left and right main bronchi. These bronchi further divide into smaller branches, called bronchioles, that are like twigs extending to the edges of the tree. The smallest unit of the lungs is the alveolus, which is where gas exchange occurs.

The diaphragm is a dome-shaped muscle that sits below the lungs and separates your chest cavity from your abdominal cavity; it is primarily responsible for ventilating air in and out of your lungs. When you breathe in, your diaphragm contracts and moves down, lowering the pressure inside your lungs. This allows air to flow into your lungs. Expiration is usually a passive process. However, if you are trying to blow air out of your lungs quickly, then your abdominal muscles and the intercostal muscles between your ribs also play a role. There are also smooth muscles surrounding the alveoli that are critical in opening your airways (i.e., bronchodilation) by relaxing when their beta-2 receptors become activated. The commonly pre-scribed rescue inhaler contains salbutamol, which activates beta-2 receptors to quickly cause bronchodilation.

If you are having trouble breathing (i.e., dyspnea), then addi-tional muscles are recruited to help with ventilation. Examples in-clude the sternocleidomastoid, upper trapezius, and scalene muscles. These muscles are in the neck, upper back, and sternum to help with inspiration. If a young child is in respiratory distress, you may notice that their head is bobbing when these muscles contract. The opening of their nose may spread wide open (i.e., nasal flaring), and you may hear grunting to help keep their lungs open. Any of these signs in children requires immediate medical attention.

The Gastrointestinal Tract

The immune system in the gastrointestinal tract maintains a delicate balance between defense against pathogens and toleration of food. It must tolerate the gut microbiome, which is the ecosystem of microorganisms that live in your gastrointestinal tract. The innate immune system is present throughout your gut because its lining acts as a physical barrier. Your stomach acid provides a first line of defense against many pathogens by directly destroying them. The adaptive immune system in the gastrointestinal tract contains gut-associated lymphoid tissue (GALT) where plasma cells produce immunoglobulin A (IgA) antibodies that help neutralize toxins and pathogens. There are regulatory T cells (Tregs) in the gut that promote tolerance of food and resident microorganisms.

Nausea and vomiting are essential defense mechanisms to help remove harmful substances such as toxins and pathogens. How does the immune system cause vomiting? There are multiple mechanisms, but mast cells are primarily involved by releasing chemicals such as histamine to trigger vomiting. This is why antihistamines such as dimenhydrinate (Dramamine), meclizine (Bonine), and promethazine (Phenergan) are used to treat nausea and vomiting.

Mast cells may also be responsible for causing diarrhea by releasing serotonin and histamine. These mediators stimulate fluid secretion into the gastrointestinal tract, contributing to diarrhea. T cell activation can also contribute to diarrhea by increasing intestinal permeability and stopping the function of certain ion channels that are responsible for sodium and water absorption, so fluid accumulates in the gastrointestinal tract.

The Skin

The largest organ in your body is saved for last in this chapter. Skin is composed of three primary layers: the epidermis, the dermis, and the hypodermis. The epidermis is the outermost layer of skin, which is composed of several sublayers. It provides a barrier against irritants, allergens, and pathogens and prevents water loss. Keratinocytes are cells in the epidermis that provide the physical barrier and produce cytokines and antimicrobial peptides that help start an immune response. Just beneath the epidermis is the dermis, which consists of hair follicles, nerves, blood vessels, and connective tissue. This layer provides structure to the skin, regulates body temperature, and provides nutrients to the skin. The hypodermis is also known as the subcutaneous layer, which contains mostly connective tissue and fat. This layer helps provide energy, insulation, and a shield against physical forces.

A type of dendritic cells in the epidermis called Langerhans cells plays a crucial role in initiating allergic reactions in the skin. These cells capture antigens and travel to local lymph nodes to activate T cells, which starts the adaptive immune response. T cells also found in the skin are known as resident memory T cells because they respond quickly to previously encountered pathogens. B cells and plasma cells are present in the skin to produce antibodies that neutralize pathogens. The immune system in your skin also interacts with nerve cells and the bacteria on your skin that may alter the immune responses.

A rash may be a sign of an underlying process driven by your immune system. Rashes are mainly divided into primary and secondary skin lesions. Primary skin lesions are changes to the skin due to an internal problem; they include macules, patches, papules, plaques, pustules, nodules, vesicles, and bullae. Macules are flat lesions that are usually less than 1 cm in diameter, while patches are larger. Papules are small, raised lesions less than 1 cm in diameter, while plaques are larger. Pustules contain pus, which is a thick, opaque fluid that contains dead white blood cells and pathogens. Nodules are larger and deeper than papules and may go into the subcutaneous layer. Vesicles are small, fluid-filled lesions that are less than 1 cm in diameter, while bullae are larger.

Secondary skin lesions are changes that occur in primary skin lesions due to external factors such as scratching or the natural progression of a disease. Examples include crusts, scales, erosions, ulcers, fissures, atrophy, and lichenification. Crusts are dried blood or pus on the surface of the skin; they are often seen after vesicles or pustules have ruptured. Scales are flakes of dead epidermal cells, which are usually due to accumulation of keratin or abnormal skin shedding. Erosions are shallow losses of epidermis that heal without scarring. These are often seen after a vesicle or bullae rupture. Ulcers are deeper losses of skin than erosions but may still heal without scarring. Fissures are cracks in the skin that may extend into the dermis, which is often seen with eczema. Atrophy is thinning of the skin, while lichenification means the skin has thickened.

I know these last couple of chapters were not necessarily the most exciting, but you should now have the foundational knowledge needed to take on the rest of this book. We can now move on to the practical clinical aspects!

TAKE-HOME POINTS

- Lymph nodes are strategically placed throughout your body to quickly respond to infections.

- The mucus that covers many of your organs helps lubricate and protect your body from pathogens.

- Your sinuses may become clogged because there is excess mucus production, impaired mucociliary clearance, and/or increased inflammation of the surrounding tissues.

CHAPTER 4

What to Expect at the Allergist's Office

Jessica was a primary school teacher who loved her students. It brought her so much joy to see her students learning. She knew she was making a difference in their lives. Jessica also had two boys at home who kept her on her toes. Despite having her hands full, she was able to run a couple of marathons each year. Jessica had some mild allergies that did not bother her unless she was around cats. As a child, she used to wheeze and her doctors labeled her with asthma, but at this point in her life, she rarely used her salbutamol inhaler unless it was prior to a long run. Jessica felt that she was healthy.

On one September day, she woke up with a fever, chills, cough, stuffy nose, and muscle aches. She was not overly concerned about it because she felt that it was a part of the job—kids pass germs all the time. However, she swabbed her nose at home and tested positive for COVID-19. She had to take off work for the rest of the week to recover and not pass the infection to her students.

At first, the symptoms felt like the flu and her fever broke after two days. She went back to work, but she felt more tired than usual for a couple of weeks. Jessica noticed that her cough never went away completely. She started using her rescue inhaler again, which helped control the cough, but she relied on the inhaler multiple times each day to get through her classes. Jessica also had a hard time breathing through her nose. She tried various cough, cold, and allergy medications that she could find at the pharmacy, but nothing seemed to give her complete relief.

After four weeks of dealing with these symptoms, Jessica had had enough. She called her doctor, who was able to squeeze her in for an office visit the next day. When she saw her doctor, they told her that she would benefit from allergy testing, so they referred her to an allergist, who happened to be me.

Navigating the healthcare system can be quite confusing, challenging, and sometimes scary. This chapter will help prepare you for a visit with an allergist. Many of the concepts covered in this chapter will also apply to navigating healthcare in general, so I believe anyone will find this chapter to be helpful.

Preparations for a Visit with an Allergist

If you need to see an allergist—or any specialist, for that manner—then you need to be prepared for the office visit. One of the most important aspects of the office visit is to be able to effectively communicate your concerns. The acronym RELIEF can be used to remember the key details for an effective office visit:

Record symptoms
Educate yourself
List medications
Identify concerns
Explain reactions
Follow advice

Record your symptoms ahead of the office visit. Create a symptom diary and keep track of the symptoms you have been experiencing.

There are several questions that may help your doctor figure out what is going on. Where is the location of the symptoms? How intense are these symptoms? When did the symptoms start? How frequent are these symptoms? How long do the symptoms last? Are there any patterns to when the symptoms start? Do the symptoms move anywhere on your body? Have you tried anything to make the symptoms better? What potentially makes the symptoms worse? Have any other doctors examined you previously? If there are any rashes, please take pictures of them multiple times to show how the rash changes over time. I know it can be difficult to take pictures while problems arise, but it can make a doctor's job a lot easier.

Spend time educating yourself on what you suspect may be going on. However, do not use Google indiscriminately, because many sources are not fully vetted, or they may cause more confusion or anxiety while you're reading about various conditions. Instead, search for information from reputable organizations. Examples include the American College of Allergy, Asthma & Immunology (ACAAI), American Academy of Allergy, Asthma & Immunology (AAAAI), Asthma and Allergy Foundation of America (AAFA), Food Allergy & Anaphylaxis Connection Team (FAACT), and the American Lung Association.

When you come to the clinic, bring a list of all current medications and supplements that you are taking. List the previous treatments you have tried as well. If you saw previous doctors, then it will be very helpful to request a transfer of medical records as early as possible. Doctors in your area may not share the same electronic medical records system, so data may need to be faxed. I work at a small private practice, and I have access to one of the local community hospitals' electronic medical records, but there are several clinics and hospitals that I do not have any access to. If the records arrive ahead of the office visit, there is a chance that your doctor may have an opportunity to review the records ahead of time, which will make the office visit more impactful. If your allergist wants you to fill out any forms, try to do this as early as possible so that time is not wasted on filling out paperwork while you are there. Do not be surprised if your allergist repeats questions that were asked on these forms. They may be trying to verify what you stated or clarify details that they want to learn more about.

Identify any concerns you have when you come for the office visit. What do you want to accomplish when you see the allergist? Are you looking for a diagnosis? A new treatment plan? When you are preparing to communicate your concerns, please do not hold back any information. Be as descriptive as possible. Explain previous reactions in as much detail as possible. The symptom diary can help jog your memory. I strongly recommend that you bring someone with you who can help advocate for you. It is easy to forget important details, and having another person with you who knows you well can help fill any memory gaps that may be crucial.

Be prepared to follow the advice of your allergist. They may order several tests, which may take multiple office visits to complete. Lifestyle changes or medications may be prescribed. Keep in mind that uncovering the correct diagnosis or most effective treatment plan may take time. It is easy to get discouraged because treatment plans may take weeks to months to show results, and testing may be inconclusive. Do not be afraid to ask questions about what your allergist thinks may be going on or why tests are being performed.

Jessica came early to her appointment with me and had all her paperwork filled out ahead of time. She did not have a symptom diary for me to review, but she was able to communicate to me her concerns. She wanted to know whether her symptoms were triggered by something that was in her environment, and she wanted a better treatment plan than what was previously prescribed by her general practitioner.

What Is Allergy Skin Testing?

When Jessica called my office to schedule an appointment, she was told that she needed to avoid antihistamine medications for several days prior to visiting with me. The reason why this is important is because antihistamine medications may interfere with allergy skin testing and cause it to become falsely negative, meaning the test will say that you do not have an allergy to a substance even though you are allergic to it. There are two primary types of allergy skin tests for food, environmental allergens, and stinging insects: percutaneous skin prick testing and intradermal testing. Each skin test relies on introducing a small amount of the allergen into the skin. If the immune system was previously sensitized to the allergen and has specific IgE antibodies that could bind to that allergen, then histamine is released when the allergen is introduced into the skin during the skin test, leading to a hive forming over where the allergen was placed. If you are taking antihistamines, then the histamine released during the test will not be able to produce a hive to indicate a positive test. Your allergist's office should tell you ahead of the appointment how long they want you to avoid medications before the testing occurs. There is another type of skin testing called patch testing that will be discussed in chapter 9.

Percutaneous skin prick testing involves introducing a small amount of allergen extract into the upper layer of skin by puncturing the skin with a drop of the allergen. The allergens for this type of test may include environmental allergens such as pollen and dust mites, food, penicillin, and stinging insect venom. There are various devices used to perform this test, and they are usually made of plastic with tiny prongs that can scratch the skin. This is usually the first test done to detect the presence of IgE antibodies. An intradermal test involves injecting a small amount of the allergen into the dermis, which is below the epidermis. This injection technique is also used for tuberculosis skin testing and vaccines such as rabies and mpox. The intradermal test may be done for environmental allergens such as pollen and pet dander, stinging insect venom or penicillin. This test usually is done if the skin prick test is negative yet the clinical suspicion remains high and the allergist does not want to potentially miss a diagnosis. Food allergens are not administered as a part of an

intradermal test because doing so does not provide significant benefit in the diagnostic process. This test also involves injecting a small
amount of food allergen under the skin with a needle, which could
get into the bloodstream and cause a severe allergic reaction. When
I test someone for food allergies, if I suspect that they have a food
allergy, I first get a skin test to help determine if there is a potential
for a reaction to occur. I also get a blood test to help track whether
there is a chance the food allergy may resolve.

Skin testing will also include a positive control that usually contains a solution of histamine to make sure the skin is properly reactive,
so you will experience itching with an allergy skin test. There will also
be a negative control that usually consists of either saline or glycerin,
which should not cause reaction in the skin testing. If there is a skin
reaction to the negative control, then the patient most likely has dermographism (see chapter 10) and the test may be impossible to interpret accurately. *Dermographism* literally means "skin writing," which
means your skin can develop hives in the areas where it is scratched.

The back and the arms are the preferred locations to place an
allergy skin test. These spots are the easiest to observe reactions
clearly while avoiding having the test extracts drip down due to
gravity. The back is slightly more reactive, but the difference is minimal. Placing the test on the arms allows the patient to see the reaction occur. Once the test is placed, it takes roughly fifteen to twenty
minutes for the immediate skin reaction to be completed. Afterward,
the extracts are wiped off and the test is interpreted. The skin test
will produce an itchy, red bump with fluid under the bump. That
fluid is referred to as a wheal and the redness around the bump is
called a flare. If the wheal is significantly larger than the negative
control test, then the test is positive.

When Jessica got her skin test, she complained that the test made
her arms feel very itchy and burning. The itching can be quite uncomfortable for some people, especially because you must sit still for a
while. Many people will spend time on their phone or reading a book
to keep their minds off the test. For young children, it can be a partic-

ularly stressful experience. Children may assume that needles will be used, which is not always the case. Check with your allergist's office ahead of time to see whether they will perform intradermal testing, and prepare the child for the visit. It is okay to tell them what may happen so that they know what to expect. Bring something that will entertain them so they can sit still. Having an extra adult accompanying you and your child may help when the test is administered.

Jessica's allergy testing was positive for pollen, cat dander, and dust mites. Afterward, topical medication was placed on her skin to help reverse the rash on her arms. Allergists may offer oral antihistamines, topical antihistamines, and/or topical steroids to treat the rash. At home, the rash may persist for several days if left untreated, so taking oral antihistamines and/or hydrocortisone 1 percent will help treat the test site. I learned this the hard way when I was in fellowship training because one of my co-fellows put a skin test on me for practice, which ended up leaving a rash that persisted for a couple of weeks!

While we do not fully understand the relationship between COVID-19, asthma, and allergies, there is some evidence to suggest that this viral infection may worsen these conditions. This is because the virus may heighten the activation of mast cells (see chapter 14). These cells may become twitchier and release chemicals such as histamine to either known allergens or nonspecific triggers such as stress, fragrances, and smoke. Jessica's immune system may not be functioning correctly in other ways, such as becoming more hypersensitive to the external environment. This may lead to additional inflammation in the airways, worsening asthma symptoms. Her recent experience with COVID-19 may be the reason why her allergy and asthma symptoms significantly worsened.

How Accurate Are Allergy Skin Tests?

Allergy skin testing is generally accurate. However, to have a better understanding of the accuracy of skin testing and medical tests in general, you need to understand the difference between the sensitivity and specificity of a test. The sensitivity of a test is the ability to correctly identify individuals who have a disease. In other words, it is the percentage of true positive results among those who have the disease. If the sensitivity of the test is 85 percent, then 85 percent of individuals with the disease will test positive and 15 percent will be false negatives. Specificity measures the ability of a test to correctly identify individuals who do not have the disease. It is the percentage of true negative results among those who do not have the disease. For example, if the specificity of a test is 90 percent, then 90 percent of those without the disease will test negative and 10 percent will be false positives. If you are screening for a diagnosis such as cancer, then you want a test with a high sensitivity. On the other hand, a confirmatory test to rule out other diagnoses would benefit from a test that has a high specificity.

Here is an analogy to highlight the difference between sensitivity and specificity. Think of sensitivity like a dog that barks when it sees an intruder. The goal is to identify an intruder through the dog's barking. If the guard dog is highly sensitive, it will bark at anything potentially suspicious such as real intruders, the mailman, or a squirrel. This means that the dog will rarely miss a real intruder (i.e., few false negatives). The downside is that the dog may bark too much and wake you up unnecessarily (i.e., false positives). On the other hand, specificity refers to the dog's ability to stay quiet unless it is a real intruder. A highly specific guard dog will bark only when it is sure that there is an intruder and will not disturb you with unnecessary barking (i.e., few false positives). However, there is a risk that the dog may miss an intruder (i.e., false negatives).

According to the AAAAI, the sensitivity and specificity of skin prick testing is generally high. A 2016 study found that the sensitivity and specificity of skin prick testing was 85 percent and 77 percent, respectively. However, if considering only food allergy skin prick testing, then the sensitivity is greater than 90 percent but the specificity is roughly 50 percent. This means that there is a higher risk of false positive results. This is why food allergy panel testing may not be beneficial for many people. Chapter 7 will discuss food allergy testing in more detail. Intradermal skin testing generally has higher sensitivity, but lower specificity compared to skin prick testing. Again, this means that this type of test is usually administered when the skin prick test is negative, yet there is a strong clinical suspicion that there is an allergy.

What Is Allergy Blood Testing?

While the skin tests indirectly measure IgE antibodies that have the potential for causing an allergic reaction, there is blood testing available that can directly measure the amount of specific IgE antibodies that can bind to an allergen. This is referred to as serum specific IgE (sIgE) testing. There are different ways to measure these antibodies. You may have heard of the radioallergosorbent (RAST) test before, but this test has been replaced with newer methods that are more accurate, such as fluorescent enzyme immunoassay (FEIA) and chemiluminescent immunoassay (CLIA). The newer tests generally involve collecting a blood sample and incubating it with the suspected allergen, which is absorbed on a solid substance such as a plastic disc or bead. The IgE antibodies are detected by adding another antibody that can bind to them and is labeled with a detectable marker such as an enzyme. Yet another type of allergy blood testing, called component-resolved diagnostics, uses purified allergens instead of crude allergen extracts and specifically looks at portions of an allergen where the IgE antibody may bind to it. This may help characterize the severity of the allergy in some cases. As an example, component testing for peanut allergy may help distinguish between a potentially severe allergy to peanuts versus a condition called oral allergy syndrome (see chapter 7 for more information).

If you have ever seen a blood allergy test, then you may have noticed that the results show an IgE level (usually measured in kU/L concentration) as well as a class number that is often listed from

0 to 5. In my opinion, looking at the class is unnecessary, because it does not provide any information that is clinically relevant. The IgE level is sufficient, because if that number is higher, then it is more likely that substance could potentially provoke an allergic reaction. The allergy blood test results can be difficult to interpret, so I highly recommend that you wait to look at these lab results until you can discuss them with your doctor.

The World Health Organization (WHO) and International Union of Immunological Societies (IUIS) created a nomenclature to describe various allergens so that people could communicate with each other about these issues. Allergen nomenclature uses the first three letters of the genus and the first letter of the species and a number to denote the order in which it was discovered. The Latin word for peanut is *Arachis hypogaea*, so an example of its allergen nomenclature looks like this—Ara h 1. The components Ara h 1, 2, 3, and 6 are associated with systemic allergic reactions, whereas Ara h 8 is associated with oral allergy syndrome.

While most health insurance plans in the United States cover allergy blood testing, they may have a preferred lab at which to get your blood drawn. Make sure you call your health insurer to verify which labs are preferred. Otherwise, it is very hard to contest the bill. While testing for one specific allergen is not very expensive, testing for multiple allergens adds up very quickly. I am glad I learned about this during my fellowship training because I could have easily seen myself accidentally ordering a series of blood tests and not disclosing this information to my patient, leaving them with an enormous medical bill.

Which Test Is More Accurate, Skin or Blood Tests?

Several studies have compared the accuracy of allergy skin testing to allergy blood testing. A study by R. L. M. Griffiths et al. found that allergy blood testing had higher rates of detecting wheat allergy than did skin testing. A study by Gabriele de Vos investigated the diagnostic accuracy of skin testing versus blood testing for environmental allergens and found that these tests cannot be used interchangeably. They believe that using only one method may misdiagnose many people. A meta-analysis by K. Soares-Weiser et al. showed that both skin and blood allergy testing for food allergies had high sensitivity but low specificity, but skin testing showed slightly higher sensitivity for certain foods such as peanuts and eggs.

In my clinical experience, I use both tests for different reasons. When a patient such as Jessica sees me for the first time, I start by performing a skin test. It is a quick test that gives you results right when you are in the clinic to tell you whether there is a potential for a substance to cause an allergic reaction. The exception is when someone accidentally takes an antihistamine medication shortly before the appointment, or they had skin testing done recently or they have dermographism. If they cannot stop their antihistamine medication or they have dermographism, then I will skip the skin testing and order blood testing. I often order blood testing when I do not have the extract for a specific allergen such as peas or lentils. If I am testing for food allergies, I will perform a skin test and order blood testing to characterize the risk level of experiencing a reaction to a potential food allergen, and then obtain blood tests over time to see whether a food allergy has resolved.

Regardless of the testing method, these tests cannot reliably predict whether a reaction to a substance will be mild or severe. The size of the wheal on a skin test or the amount of specific IgE antibody measured in a blood test only tells us how likely a reaction may be. There are several other factors that cannot be measured from these tests that may dictate the severity of an allergic reaction. Examples include poorly controlled asthma, fever, and exercise.

Ways to Advocate for Yourself While at the Office

Let's get back to Jessica. She had skin testing that found potential environmental triggers for her symptoms. It appeared that her asthma had returned based on lung function testing that was obtained and that she needed a new inhaler for daily use (see chapter 11). I asked her if she knew how to use an inhaler, and she told me she had been using one on and off for many years and felt comfortable she knew how to use it. However, when I asked her to show me how to use it, she made several mistakes. If you are prescribed an inhaler medication, make sure you ask your doctor and/or pharmacist how to use it. This is especially important for allergic diseases such as asthma and food allergy where medications may require multiple steps to use them correctly. I gave Jessica a written asthma action plan to explain what medications should be taken based on her symptoms. Ask your doctor to have a written treatment plan that you can refer to when you need guidance on what to do.

Do not be afraid to ask specific questions about your health and the treatment plan. Before a test, you may ask, Why is the test being done? How is the test performed? How long does the test take? Are there any risks to this test? If a diagnosis is made, then you may want to ask about how the condition is treated. Ask about the risks and benefits of the treatments or management plans that are being offered to you. Will the condition go away? What resources are available to learn more?

There may be times when it is not clear what is going on, and this can be extemely difficult. Unfortunately, doctors may not be able to diagnose every condition the first time they see you. The human body is incredibly complex, and many symptoms can overlap with different diseases. If you are struggling to know what is going on, one of the most important questions to ask your doctor is this: What do you think is the differential diagnosis for me? *Differential diagnosis* is a term used in healthcare to describe the list of possible conditions that could explain someone's symptoms. The process that doctors use to diagnose and treat diseases is rooted in the scientific method, which is a systematic, logical approach to solving problems. It starts with making an observation that generates a question or identifies a problem. Information is gathered that leads to a hypothesis, which is an educated guess. The hypothesis is then tested, and data is collected and analyzed. Based on the results, the hypothesis is either accepted or rejected. If the hypothesis is rejected, then a new hypothesis and testing are started to try and answer the original question.

A doctor gathers information about their patient through taking a detailed history. What is the problem that brings them into the clinic (i.e., chief complaint)? What are the details of the issues they are dealing with? What are their previous medical problems? Is there a family history of any diseases? Are there any allergies to medications? What medications are they taking? These questions narrow the differential diagnosis, which is fine-tuned by a physical examination. The doctor has prior experience and knowledge of various diseases and their underlying mechanisms (i.e., pathophysiology) to then generate the differential diagnosis. This is not often communicated with their patients, which is why it is so important for you to ask them what they are thinking could be going on. Once that differential diagnosis is created, testing will be ordered to help narrow the possibilities further. The initial hypothesis the doctor makes is what the most likely diagnosis is that explains the patient's symptoms based on all the information collected. A treatment plan is prescribed and then the patient needs to be followed closely to determine whether the initial diagnosis and treatment were correct. If the plan does not work, then additional information and possible testing need to be obtained to determine a new diagnosis and treatment plan.

Jessica was given a new treatment plan that focused on reducing exposure to her allergens and updating her asthma medications. She needed to take an asthma maintenance inhaler that contained a small amount of steroid to reduce the inflammation in her lungs. She also started a daily nasal spray that contained a steroid. Over the course of a few weeks, she felt significantly better and was able to start running again.

While we know a lot about the human body, there is much more that we need to learn about it. There are diseases that we do not fully understand, or there are no tests available to identify easily what is going on. As an example, chapter 14 dives into mast cell disorders that are quite challenging to diagnose and manage. And chapter 18, the last chapter of this book, will introduce you to where research is going in treating various allergic diseases. This will give you a sense of how much we need to learn. While I strongly encourage you to stick with a doctor for a few visits, if you feel that you are not being heard or you are not satisfied, then it is fine to get a second opinion from another doctor.

Now that you have all the background information relating to anatomy, immunology, and navigating healthcare, it is time to get into more information relating to allergic disease.

TAKE-HOME POINTS

- Be prepared for your appointment with your allergist by keeping a symptom diary, bringing an additional family member, and avoiding medications as instructed by your doctor's office.

- Allergy skin and blood testing are both helpful for evaluating allergic diseases. Both may be used for different reasons.

- If you are struggling to find answers for what is causing your symptoms, it may take multiple visits over time. Seek a second opinion if you are not satisfied.

Part Two

Allergic Diseases

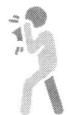 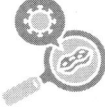 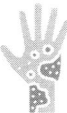

CHAPTER 5

Allergic Rhinitis and Non-Allergic Rhinitis

R obert was a successful businessman and dedicated athlete who led a life that demanded mental and physical sharpness. Even in his sixties, he did not feel the need to slow down. Robert spent his days running long distances in the morning, followed by a flurry of meetings and presentations. However, throughout his entire life, he had silently struggled with various symptoms. Every morning, he woke up with a stuffy nose and itchy eyes, and had sneezing fits throughout the day. He had a difficult time concentrating at work or finishing his workouts as fast as he wanted. Robert tried every over-the-counter medication you could think of, such as Claritin, Benadryl, and Flonase, but his symptoms persisted.

When he felt particularly bad, he lost focus at work, which sometimes coincided with important business meetings. Robert tried to hide his symptoms from his colleagues because he did not want to appear weak or be a distraction. He was frustrated that he could never find complete relief from his allergies. However, one of Robert's closest friends at work realized that he was struggling and encouraged him to see an allergist to help get his symptoms under control.

What Is Allergic Rhinitis and Non-Allergic Rhinitis?

Rhinitis is inflammation of the nasal passages that manifests as at least one of the following symptoms: stuffy nose (nasal congestion), runny nose (rhinorrhea), postnasal drip, sneezing, or nasal itching. These symptoms, which may include itchy, red or pink eyes, swollen eyelids, and tearing, are often associated with conjunctivitis. The underlying mechanism of rhinitis is what distinguishes allergic rhinitis from non-allergic rhinitis. Allergic rhinitis has several names, including hay fever, nasal allergies, and seasonal allergies, or just allergies. When the symptoms occur during only part of the year, it is known as seasonal allergic rhinitis, and when the symptoms occur year-round, it is known as perennial allergic rhinitis. For the sake of decreasing confusion, I will stick to saying allergic rhinitis throughout this book. In this case, the inflammation that leads to allergic rhinitis is due to the creation of IgE antibodies that can specifically bind to allergens such as pollen, mold, pet dander, dust mites, and more. If there is no evidence that these allergic triggers are causing the symptoms, then the condition is usually called non-allergic rhinitis. There are other terms used to describe non-allergic rhinitis, including vasomotor rhinitis, intrinsic rhinitis, and idiopathic rhinitis. I will also discuss other distinct types of rhinitis, but in general, I will use the term non-allergic rhinitis throughout this book.

Regardless of the underlying mechanism, rhinitis causes significant health problems. Up to 30 percent of Americans have allergic rhinitis. One of the greatest problems associated with uncontrolled rhinitis is sleep disturbances. One in four adults reported that they either cannot sleep or are awakened most nights due to their symptoms. Up to half of adults reported that allergic rhinitis has at least a moderate effect on their daily life. Some people who have rhinitis have a decreased sense of smell, which makes it more difficult to properly taste and enjoy food. Allergic rhinitis is also associated with attention deficit hyperactivity disorder, anxiety, depression, lower exam scores, reduced athletic performance, and lower self-esteem. There is also a higher risk of developing sinus infections and ear infections. Asthma symptoms may worsen if the underlying triggers are due to environmental allergens.

Rhinitis puts an enormous burden on society. The medical costs of allergic rhinitis in the United States are between $3 billion and $4 billion annually. Multiple studies have reported that people living with allergic rhinitis miss between one and ten workdays per year. This is not just an American problem. Allergic rhinitis sickens roughly 40 percent of people living in Japan and was declared a "national disease" by Prime Minister Fumio Kishida in 2023. Twenty percent of Japanese companies offer remote work options during their pollen season because over $1.5 billion is lost daily in Japan due to missed workdays and decreased productivity. The IT company Aisaac offers a "tropical escape" program that allows employees to move to anywhere with low pollen levels from mid-February through mid-April. The most common domestic destinations are Okinawa and Amami Oshima, but some people move to Guam or Hawaii. Aisaac also pays their employees up to $1,300 for this program.

Why Is Allergic Rhinitis Becoming More Common?

Every spring, I see many new patients who are either recently starting to have trouble with allergic rhinitis for the first time or their symptoms have significantly worsened compared to the previous year. Patients ask me constantly, "Why are my allergies worse than ever before?" The answer to this question is still under investigation, but I will address some of the hypotheses.

The genetics that you inherit from your parents can increase the risk of developing allergic rhinitis and other allergic diseases.

However, the rapid rise in these diseases is not due to genetic mutations alone. There must be environmental and/or lifestyle factors driving the allergy epidemic. You may have heard of the *hygiene hypothesis*, a term coined by epidemiologist David Strachan in 1989. This hypothesis proposes that fewer infections in childhood could explain the rise in allergic diseases. Over time, the hygiene hypothesis has taken on different meanings, including the idea that we have become too clean and that early childhood infections are important for regulating the immune system. Even though vaccines and antibiotics have decreased the burden of infectious diseases, hygiene is still important in the twenty-first century. Hygiene is the first line of defense when new threats emerge, such as a new influenza strain, Ebola, and SARS-CoV-2 (the virus that causes COVID-19), before vaccines are available. Antibiotic resistance has become a global threat, and hygiene helps reduce the spread of bacteria in the community and in hospitals.

Infections can increase the risk of developing cancer or other chronic diseases. Various strains of human papillomavirus (HPV) are associated with developing cervical cancer. Epstein-Barr virus infection is a major contributing factor to developing multiple sclerosis. Rhinovirus and respiratory syncytial virus (RSV) have been associated with developing asthma later in life. SARS-CoV-2 is also associated with developing or worsening various allergic diseases, including allergic rhinitis and asthma. In fact, the lockdowns that occurred in 2020 to help slow the spread of COVID-19 may have helped reduce the risk of babies developing various allergic diseases. Multiple studies from Europe confirm that childhood infections do not protect against allergic diseases.

The Old Friends mechanism, proposed by Graham Rook in 2003, builds upon the hygiene hypothesis by arguing that the vital exposures during childhood are not to childhood infections such as the common cold or chickenpox. Instead, early exposure to other relatively harmless microbes that colonize the skin, gut, and respiratory tract may be vital to properly regulating the immune system.

Multiple epidemiologic studies reported that cesarean section may increase the risk of developing allergic diseases since infants are not exposed to microbes in the vaginal canal. Breast milk may play a role in reducing the risk of developing allergic diseases since it is not sterile. More studies are needed to fully understand the role of microorganisms in developing allergic diseases.

The reason that rhinitis is increasing may be far more obvious. One of the most common culprits for triggering seasonal allergies is pollen, which is tiny grains produced as a part of the sexual reproductive cycle of many plants, including trees, grasses, and ragweed. Pollen counts have been steadily increasing over the years, but why has this been happening?

There is one hypothesis that does not hold much weight, but the concept goes viral on social media every spring: *botanical sexism*. Horticulturalist Thomas Ogren coined the term, and his ideas have been featured in *Scientific American* and on NPR. The idea sounds sensible on the surface: Ogren argued that the reason allergies are worse now is because city planners purposely planted only male trees, which produce pollen. Over time, pollen counts would continually rise because of a scarcity of female trees. In his op-ed in *Scientific American* in 2015, he referenced the 1949 USDA *Yearbook of Agriculture*, which said, "When used for street plantings, only male trees should be selected, to avoid the nuisance from cottony seed." However, there is no conspiracy here. This passage was specifically referring to cottonwood trees, not male trees in general. The next sentence in this passage stated, "Roots of the cottonwood often clog sewer and drain pipes. The wood is weak and subject to breaking in storms." The problem with the botanical sexism hypothesis is that most trees are not specifically male or female. Most trees have both male and female reproductive organs.

Even though botanical sexism probably does not explain why pollen counts are increasing, this problem is still most likely self-inflicted. Since humans have been burning fossil fuels, we have been adding carbon dioxide to the atmosphere, which is a greenhouse gas that has been warming the globe. The pollen season has been lasting longer since there are fewer days with below freezing temperatures each year. Carbon dioxide is an important nutrient for plants, and multiple studies have reported that pollen counts have been rising as carbon dioxide levels rise. Researchers in South Korea planted oak trees in September 2009 that were in special chambers where they could control the carbon dioxide levels. The amount of carbon dioxide exposure was increased to the projected levels for 2050. Then they measured the pollen counts in 2018 and found that there was an increase in pollen grain production per tree of 353 to 1,299 percent compared to trees exposed to the current carbon dioxide levels. In addition, the pollen grains contained more proteins on the outer shell of the pollen, so the immune system has more opportunities to create an allergic reaction. This means that not only have greenhouse gas emissions caused pollen seasons to last longer, but the seasons are also becoming more severe. Recent projections predict that by the year 2100, pollen season may start ten to forty days earlier and end five to fifteen days later. The amount of pollen released may be 40 percent higher as well. We will have to make some serious systemic changes in climate policy to help our future generations be able to breathe cleaner air.

What Are the Triggers of Allergic Rhinitis and Non-Allergic Rhinitis?

Robert had a dog named Daisy who would go running with him. While he usually did not have more symptoms around Daisy, if she licked him, then he would feel itchy and have a sneezing attack. Daisy also slept in his bedroom at the foot of his bed. Sometimes, she would jump in between Robert and his wife when there was a rainstorm.

"Daisy is a Goldendoodle, so she is hypoallergenic. I have worse symptoms around other dogs," Robert told me.

He could never be around cats because his chest would feel tight when he was near one. Almost 10 million Americans are allergic to their pets. Both cats and dogs have proteins in their saliva, skin cells (i.e., dander), and urine that can cause allergic reactions. Hypoallergenic dog and cat breeds are a myth. While these animals make varying amounts of allergens, we cannot reliably predict which breeds produce fewer allergens. Researchers have measured dog allergens in dust samples from homes that have dogs and have not found any significant difference in the amount of allergens present based on dog breeds classified as "hypoallergenic." It does not matter whether the animals shed, or the length of their hair or fur. I wish we had a reliable way to predict which animals shed fewer allergens, but we do not have that capability right now.

Plants release pollen every spring, summer, and fall. The plants that cause allergic rhinitis are trees, grasses, and weeds that spread pollen in the air in massive quantities. In the United States, tree pollen is typically released from February through May. Examples include oak, maple, beech, birch, walnut, ash, elm, juniper, and cottonwood. Grass pollen is released from April through June: Bahia, Bermuda, Johnson grass, fescue, timothy, and Kentucky blue are common grasses that cause allergic rhinitis. Weed pollen is released from July through October and includes ragweed, lamb's-quarters, mugwort, pigweed, and Russian thistle. However, in some southern states such as Texas and Oklahoma, tree pollen season starts as early as December. This is because mountain cedar trees start to release a massive amount of pollen in the winter that leads to a condition known as cedar fever. Since many people start having allergy symptoms during the typical cold and flu season, people find it difficult to determine whether their symptoms are due to allergic rhinitis, the common cold, influenza, or COVID-19. The symptoms are similar among these illnesses, but allergic rhinitis does not cause a fever, and itching does not commonly occur with influenza or COVID-19.

When I asked Robert about his home environment, he told me he lived in a home that is over a century old. The home exudes a quaint charm, with its original hardwood floors and vintage moldings, which takes you back to the roaring twenties. However, the home is very dusty, and Robert is concerned that it may be contaminated with mold, which is fungi that grow in multicellular filaments called hyphae. Mold can come in various colors, including green, black, white, blue, orange, and yellow. Mildew is a type of mold growth that is usually flat. The mold spores that are released in the air primarily cause allergy symptoms. Mold can grow in damp environments. The usual places you may find mold in your home include the kitchen, bathroom, attic, basement, windowsills, and HVAC system. Mold also grows on rotting logs, compost piles, grasses, and fallen leaves. While not all molds cause allergy symptoms, the most common ones that do include penicillium, Alternaria, Cladosporium, and aspergillus. Symptoms can occur year-round due to mold found indoors, but mold allergies can be most severe from July through the first hard frost of the year because of mold spores inhaled while outside.

A component of dust that causes significant allergy symptoms is dust mites. These eight-legged creatures include *Dermatophagoides pteronyssinus*, *Dermatophagoides farinae*, *Euroglyphus maynei*, and *Blomia tropicalis*. They are pale, translucent, and do not have eyes! Dust mites are the size of the tip of a very sharp pencil, so while they are technically large enough to be visible to the naked eye, dust mites usually cannot be seen because they are translucent and are afraid of the light. Their droppings are what causes allergy symptoms. Dust mite allergen levels are higher in homes that are older and do not have air-conditioning. Flats in the inner city have lower dust mite counts, but they have higher mouse and cockroach allergens. In homes, dust mites are primarily found where there are skin cells, high humidity, and low light. This includes bedding, pillows, mattresses, carpets, curtains, stuffed animals, upholstered furniture, and dusty areas. While dust mites may be found in feathered pillows, there are more allergens found in synthetic pillows. Dust mites can also colonize wheat products and pet food.

Non-allergic triggers are numerous, but there are several important examples. Strong fragrances and scents can be irritating to the nasal passages and lead to rhinitis. Any kind of smoking, whether it is from tobacco products, a hookah, or vaping may not only cause coughing but also nasal symptoms. Quitting smoking and avoiding secondhand exposure is the best way to prevent these symptoms. Weather changes, such as fluctuations in barometric pressure, humidity, and temperature can affect people. Some people experience a runny nose or sneezing after eating hot or spicy foods, which is referred to as gustatory rhinitis. The milk-mucus effect is the belief that drinking milk increases mucus production and worsens nasal congestion. However, there is not much scientific evidence that this phenomenon is due to an abnormal immune response. Milk has a creamy texture, which can coat the roof of the mouth and throat and trick the senses into believing that there is more mucus production.

The hormonal changes that occur during pregnancy may also cause rhinitis. About a third of women report that their symptoms worsen during pregnancy while another third report that their symptoms improve. Unfortunately, pregnancy rhinitis does not respond well to medications. Regular exercise may help by causing blood vessels in the nasal passages to constrict. Nasal dilator strips help open the nasal passages temporarily. Elevating the head of the bed by 30 to 45 degrees helps the nasal passages drain more effectively while sleeping. Rinsing the nasal passages with saline water may help as well.

Testing for Allergic Rhinitis and Non-Allergic Rhinitis

Susan worked for a start-up company that was using 3D printing to build its products. She dealt with allergic rhinitis that mainly occurred in the spring throughout her childhood, but after she had kids, her symptoms became year-round. She experienced sneezing attacks at work and at home. It became so distracting at work that coworkers nicknamed her "Sneezing Suzie." At night, she could barely breathe through her nose, which made sleeping difficult. Susan had two dogs and a cat at home that were inseparable from her children.

Nothing she took over the counter relieved her symptoms completely, so she came to see me to get an allergy test. Susan told me that at work, whenever the 3D printer was running, her symptoms were worse. Her physical examination was notable for dark circles under her eyes, called allergic shiners. This is a sign that her nose was chronically congested. She also had small folds under her eyelids that are called Dennie-Morgan lines, which look like wrinkles, but they are a sign of rhinitis or eczema, not aging. The back of her throat had little bumps resembling cobblestones. Susan told me that she cleared her throat throughout the day, which is a sign of mucus draining in the back of her throat (i.e., postnasal drip). Her nasal turbinates were enlarged and pale, which means that the nasal passages may have allergic inflammation.

Keep in mind that not all noses are stuffy because of allergic or non-allergic rhinitis. There could be chronic rhinosinusitis with or without nasal polyps, which will be discussed more in the next chapter. The septum, which separates the nostrils, can deviate and make it harder to breathe through one of the nostrils. There could be a foreign body such as a bead or pea that is stuck in a nostril. Tumors can be found in the nasal passages as well. Children with recurrent ear infections and/or snoring may have an enlarged adenoid tissue in the back of the throat. This is why it is so important to have a doctor check into all potential causes for rhinitis.

As previously mentioned in chapter 4, the two main types of allergy tests are skin tests and blood tests. Susan got a skin test that was positive for cats, dogs, dust mites, and tree pollen. Because her symptoms were worse at work around the 3D printer, I suspected that she was also sensitive to chemicals used during the 3D printing process. Volatile organic compounds are gases that can be emitted during 3D printing and can irritate the lungs and nasal passages when inhaled. When nasal symptoms occur in the workplace from sources that are not normally seen outside the workplace, this is often referred to as occupational rhinitis. The gold standard for proving there is a problem in the workplace is to perform a procedure called a direct nasal challenge. This is when you expose someone to a small amount of the substance you suspect they are sensitive to and record their symptoms and laboratory parameters such as nasal airway resistance. Specialized rhinomanometry equipment is used for these nasal challenges. Unfortunately, this type of testing is mostly available only in research settings because it requires specialized training, and it is expensive. For Susan, her symptoms became much better controlled when she reduced her exposure to the chemicals at work and started using nasal saline rinses and a nasal steroid every day.

Management and Treatment Options

Robert's allergy testing was positive for dogs, mold, and dust mites. In cases like his, management involves medications, allergen immunotherapy, and reducing exposure to allergens or irritants. Chapter 15 will go into more details surrounding the medications used to treat allergic and non-allergic rhinitis. However, it is important to recognize that oral antihistamine medications do not work as well for non-allergic rhinitis, but nasal sprays containing antihistamines may be helpful. Rinsing the sinuses with saline water can help any form of rhinitis by removing mucus, allergens, and irritants from the nasal passages. This helps nasal sprays to become more effective since the medication will make more direct contact with tissue instead of with snot. Do not use straight tap water. It could potentially cause a severe infection! Instead, use either sterile water, distilled water, or previously boiled and cooled tap water. Chapter 16 will discuss allergen immunotherapy, which can help treat the underlying allergic immune response. Unfortunately, allergen immunotherapy is not available for non-allergic rhinitis. The remainder of this chapter will discuss allergen avoidance.

For allergen avoidance measures to be successful, there must be multiple interventions done regularly. I want to pay special attention to this because it can be extensive and there usually is not enough time available to go over these concepts in a doctor's office.

Since the COVID-19 pandemic, there has been a better appreciation of the benefits of masking. When it comes to reducing allergen exposure while outside, when using public transportation, in indoor spaces with poor air ventilation, or while you are cleaning, wearing a KN95 or N95 mask can significantly reduce exposure to allergens. The size of allergen particles is measured by their diameter in micrometers (µm). A pollen grain is typically 30 µm, dust mite allergens are roughly 20 µm, mold spores range from 2 to 40 µm, and cat allergens range from 1 to 20 µm. To give you more context, the diameter of the period at the end of a sentence is roughly 400 µm. Allergens are often attached to larger particles such as water, so a well-fitted KN95 or N95 mask can effectively filter most allergens.

The bedroom is one of the most important places in the home for reducing allergen exposure because that is where most people spend most of their time in their homes. Your immune system has a circadian rhythm and operates differently at night while you sleep, so you may be more susceptible to allergens during this important resting period. I am not a fan of carpets because they trap various indoor allergens. Removing carpets in favor of polished floors is ideal. If that is not possible, then vacuuming at least once or twice a week helps keep allergens low. Encase mattresses and pillows with covers that contain plastic or impermeable fabric to reduce dust mite allergens. Wash bedding at least once weekly at 60°C. If you straighten your bed immediately when you wake up, then you may trap moisture in the bedding and increase dust mite allergens. Wait a few hours before making your bed so the moisture dries out more effectively. Reducing indoor relative humidity to below 50 percent will help reduce dust mite and mold allergens. If there is mold identified in your home, then you may need to hire a professional for removal.

Pest management can help prevent and reduce exposure to cockroach and rodent allergens. Seal as many access points to the house as possible. Cleaning regularly and enclosing all food sources will help prevent an accumulation of allergens. Spraying insecticides releases volatile organic compounds that can irritate the nasal passages and respiratory tract, so this may not be a great option.

Robert had no intention of removing his dog from his home, and I had no intention of even suggesting this. Daisy is a part of his family! There are ways to help reduce animal allergens, including vacuuming regularly, using HEPA air purifiers, and bathing the animal regularly (although bathing cats is very difficult!). Animals should not be sleeping in your bedroom because that leads to prolonged exposure. Wash your hands and face after playing with an animal.

Cat allergens are more difficult to clean than dog allergens because they are not only tiny particles but are also very sticky. Even if a cat is removed from the home, cat allergens can linger for many months. In fact, analysis of dust from a NASA space shuttle found measurable quantities of cat allergen, but no dust mites were found! One treatment that is available only for cats is a food specifically designed to reduce the major allergenic protein in a cat's saliva, called Fel d 1. This protein is spread to their hair and dander when they groom themselves. Purina developed Pro Plan LiveClear, a food that contains an IgY antibody that neutralizes Fel d 1 in the cat's saliva. This antibody is produced by chickens when they are immunized with Fel d 1 and is passed into the yolk of their eggs. This egg yolk is added to the cat food. After cats have consumed this food daily for about three to four weeks, their Fel d 1 levels are reduced by 47 percent on average. I have seen people on social media talk about sprinkling egg yolk onto other cat food to try to reproduce these results. The problem with that approach is that you do not know whether the eggs are sourced from chickens that were exposed to cats long enough to produce enough neutralizing antibodies.

Pollen counts rise after dew dries and usually peak by midday and then fall in the evening. When the weather is hot, dry, and windy, the pollen counts tend to be higher than on days when it is raining. Keeping windows and doors closed during pollen season and having a HEPA filter in your air-conditioning unit helps reduce the amount of pollen entering your home. If you have been outside, keep your shoes in one area of the house and change your clothing immediately. Bathing at nighttime will help wash off the allergens on your body.

I'll share a quick personal story, one that illustrates some of the misinformation out there. When I interviewed for allergy fellowship training programs, I went to New York and stayed with my aunt. After she picked me up from the airport, she told me that she was very excited about my future profession.

"Tell your patients that eating local honey can help treat their allergies!" my aunt told me. At that time, I had never heard of that treatment option for allergic rhinitis. Later, during my fellowship training, I realized that this was a myth. The concept is that there is a small amount of pollen in honey that, when ingested daily, may act like allergen immunotherapy and train the immune system to become less reactive to pollen. While honey can be used for people age twelve months and older for a sore throat and cough, any pollen that is present is unlikely to be from wind-pollinated plants. The pollen that may be found in honey is from insect-pollinated plants. These pollen grains are not found in the air in large quantities, so you are not exposed to this type of pollen regularly. Any time you sneeze when smelling pretty flowers, such as roses, this is likely from the fragrance and not the pollen grains. This is another example of non-allergic rhinitis. Honey can be a tasty treat, but it is not an effective treatment for allergic rhinitis.

Ultimately, both allergic rhinitis and non-allergic rhinitis can lead to frustrating symptoms that can disrupt daily life. Whether triggered by pollen, pet dander, or environmental irritants, both allergic and non-allergic rhinitis are abnormal responses by the immune system and lead to similar symptoms. Understanding the difference between these two diseases is key to finding effective treatment strategies, from allergen avoidance and medications to immunotherapy.

TAKE-HOME POINTS

- While allergic rhinitis and non-allergic rhinitis present as similar symptoms, the underlying mechanisms and treatments differ.

- Rising pollen counts are likely happening due to rising global temperatures and increased greenhouse gas emissions.

- Treatment involves reducing exposure to the underlying triggers, taking medications, and potentially using allergen immunotherapy.

CHAPTER 6

Sinusitis

Steven woke up early one frigid morning for a workout before school and noticed a slight scratchiness in his throat and a dull ache behind his eyes. He brushed off these symptoms, thinking they were because he stayed up late the night before, doing homework. His pain subsided after he took a warm shower. However, when Steven arrived at school, pressure started to build up in his face. He felt like there was something stuck in his nose, but he could not get anything out when he tried to blow it. He started getting headaches in his forehead and cheeks that intensified as the day wore on. The pain was so severe that Steven struggled to focus while at school and at football practice.

Two weeks later, his symptoms were still present. He was not sleeping well at night, and he was fatigued throughout the day. Steven's sense of smell became diminished, and he was not able to enjoy his favorite foods—they tasted bland. His parents were frustrated that he was not feeling better, so they took Steven to his pediatrician, and he was diagnosed with sinusitis.

What Is Acute Sinusitis?

The paranasal sinuses are usually sterile. These cavities produce mucus that exits the sinuses into the nasal passages through small holes called ostia. Viruses, bacteria, and fungi are normally cleared from the sinus and nasal cavities by a process called mucociliary clearance. Think of this process as a factory conveyor belt that is lined with sticky flypaper. Mucus is like the paper, trapping germs and debris that are then moved along by the cilia, hairlike projections that are like the conveyor belt, keeping the germs from infecting the body, either by ingesting them and letting stomach acid destroy them or by inducing coughing and sneezing that push the germs out of the body. Recently, scientists have discovered that there are particles, called extracellular vesicles, that act as decoys for germs to attack instead of the lining of your nasal cavity. When the temperature and humidity drop, these extracellular vesicles and mucociliary clearance are disrupted, which increases the risk of developing an infection.

Sinusitis and *rhinosinusitis* are synonymous terms describing inflammation in the paranasal sinuses. These terms are used interchangeably because inflammation in the paranasal sinuses is almost always accompanied by inflammation in the nasal cavity. If you ever get a chance to hear an allergist or ear, nose, and throat (ENT) surgeon talk about rhinosinusitis, it sounds really confusing because the terminology is long, and even the acronyms are long. I will show you what the usual medical terminology is, but I will try to simplify the terms as much as possible. Instead of *rhinosinusitis*, I will shorten it to *sinusitis* throughout this chapter.

When symptoms occur for less than twelve weeks, it is considered acute sinusitis, which affects about 15 percent of Americans each year. When I talk about acute sinusitis, I am going to drop the term *acute* to simplify the name. The most common cause of this condition is an upper respiratory infection from a virus. A complication of viral sinusitis is a secondary bacterial infection. There are several reasons this may happen. For example, the initial damage that a viral infection can cause may help make it easier for bacteria to invade. Also, viruses may suppress certain functions of the immune system that are necessary to protect against bacteria. Roughly 6 to 9 percent of viral upper respiratory infections in children develop into bacterial sinusitis. The most common bacteria that infect the sinuses include *Streptococcus pneumoniae*, *Haemophilus influenzae*, *Moraxella catarrhalis*, and *Staphylococcus aureus*. These infections can occur at any age, even in infants occasionally. Younger children are less likely to be diagnosed with bacterial sinusitis because an ear infection is more likely to develop first, which is normally treated with antibiotics before sinusitis develops; and the sinus ostia are relatively larger compared to older children's, so the sinuses are less likely to get clogged.

There are many risk factors for developing sinusitis. For young children, day-care attendance is an important risk factor since there is a higher chance of developing a viral upper respiratory infection compared to other children. Older age, swimming, smoking, dental disease, asthma, allergic rhinitis, and changes in atmospheric pressure due to deep-sea diving and air travel are other common risk factors. Some people may have an anatomical obstruction that predisposes them to sinusitis such as a deviated nasal septum, enlarged adenoids, masses, or polyps. A primary immune deficiency disease may increase the risk of developing sinusitis as well.

Understanding the difference between viral and bacterial sinusitis is crucial because viral sinusitis typically resolves between seven and fourteen days and does not need antibiotics. We do not want to overuse antibiotics because it can increase the risk of developing antibiotic-resistant bacteria. On the other hand, untreated bacterial sinusitis may develop severe complications. They are rare, but bacteria may spread to other areas and cause swelling that includes around the eye (periorbital cellulitis), behind the eye (orbital cellulitis), in the bones (osteomyelitis), and in the brain (e.g., meningitis, intracranial abscess). A blood clot may also form in the cavernous sinuses, which is the space behind the eyes and under the brain (i.e., cavernous sinus thrombosis).

A cough, nasal symptoms including runny nose, postnasal drip, and nasal congestion, as well as a sore throat can occur with either a viral upper respiratory infection or viral sinusitis. The nasal mucus can change in color and quality as the illness progresses. It can become thicker and appear yellow or green. However, it is a myth that yellow or green snot means you need antibiotics, because it does not necessarily indicate that there is a bacterial infection occurring.

Let's review what the color of snot possibly means. If your snot is clear, this could be totally normal or possibly due to allergic or non-allergic rhinitis. White snot may be a sign of an infection, usually the common cold. During an infection, inflamed nasal tissues slow the flow of mucus, and the loss of moisture leads to the snot becoming thick and cloudy. Yellow or green mucus is a possible sign that you have an infection. White blood cells that are fighting off an infection release various waste products that change color to yellow or green. Red or pink snot means blood. When the blood is old, it turns orange or brown. Black snot could be a sign of a fungal infection or inhalation of debris, smoke, or chemicals. These colors cannot help us differentiate between viral and bacterial infection, which is why the color of snot is not a requirement for diagnosing bacterial sinusitis.

There are typically three scenarios to look for when considering whether someone may have bacterial sinusitis, which I will illustrate through some short stories:

1. Seth caught a cold from his younger sister, Sarah. For over ten days, he battled a constant feeling of a blocked nose and a persistent cough that was worse at night. His snot varied from watery to thick and yellow. His symptoms were persistent and showed no signs of improvement.

2. When four-year-old Jane woke up feeling warm and irritable, her parents initially thought it was just another cold. However, her temperature spiked to 103°F and she had a fever for three days straight. Her nose was flowing with a thick, green discharge. Jane was breathing comfortably, but her symptoms remained mostly unchanged.

3. Anne seemed to be on the mend after spending a week with what her parents thought was a typical cold. Her energy was returning as her cough got better and she was sleeping well at night. However, on the eighth day of her illness, her symptoms took a sharp turn in the wrong direction. She complained of a pounding headache, she developed a fever, and she became exhausted. This is what some doctors refer to as a "double sickening."

Imaging studies such as CT and MRI are not generally needed for sinusitis unless there is a concern that there is a potential complication such as those mentioned previously. Usually, bacterial sinusitis can be treated without testing. However, if there are concerns that the initial therapy is not working, or there are recurrent episodes of bacterial sinusitis, the person is immunocompromised, or there are other potential complications, then a specialist may want to identify the pathogen by taking a sample directly from the sinuses.

What Is Chronic Sinusitis?

For years, Sam struggled to breathe through his nose, and he felt a constant dull pressure behind his eyes that never seemed to go away. He thought this was just seasonal allergies and tried every over-the-counter medication, but his symptoms never seemed to improve. Slowly, he noticed that his sense of smell was fading. Sam was not able to enjoy food like he used to because everything started to taste bland. He was clearing his throat every day because he had this constant feeling that mucus was traveling down the back of his throat.

If you were to sit in on a lecture at a university about chronic rhinosinusitis (CRS), the slides would have two confusing acronyms. Chronic rhinosinusitis with nasal polyps would be written as CRSwNP and chronic rhinosinusitis without nasal polyps would be written as CRSsNP. I think it is less confusing if it is written as CRS with nasal polyps or without nasal polyps, which is how it will be written for this chapter.

CRS is considered when someone is experiencing symptoms that resemble sinusitis for twelve weeks or longer. Symptoms generally need to be two of the following: facial pain, pressure, or fullness; nasal blockage or congestion; nasal drainage; reduction of the sense of smell. There are multiple risk factors for developing CRS and associated conditions. Most patients with CRS have allergic rhinitis and they are usually sensitive to perennial allergens such as dust mites, mold, pet dander, and cockroaches. Roughly one in five people living with CRS have asthma, and many of these individuals experience symptoms of depression. Sustained exposure to air pollution and smoking are significant risk factors for developing CRS. Cystic fibrosis (CF) and primary ciliary dyskinesia are diseases highly associated with CRS because they cause impaired mucociliary clearance. CRS may also be a feature of systemic diseases that cause inflammation of the blood vessels (i.e., vasculitis), such as granulomatosis with polyangiitis (formerly known as Wegener's granulomatosis) or eosinophilic granulomatosis with polyangiitis (formerly known as Churg-Strauss vasculitis). Keep in mind that these diseases involve symptoms from multiple organ systems, and they are rare diseases.

CRS may be associated with nasal polyps, which are translucent, glistening, gelatinous masses that are yellowish gray to white. They look almost like shriveled grapes if they were translucent. Inside, nasal polyps contain inflammatory material that may form in the sinuses or nasal cavity. Roughly 1 to 4 percent of the population has nasal polyps. We do not fully understand why CRS and nasal polyps develop. Infections are probably a significant underlying cause of CRS, especially if no polyps are present. Or CRS may be the result of the immune system staying in a chronic inflammatory state after an infection resolves. Think of the body's immune response like a construction crew repairing a road after a flood. Normally, the crew patches things up and then leaves once the road is repaired. However, in a chronic inflammatory state such as CRS, it's as if the construction crew keeps working on the road, continually digging and redoing work that is unnecessary. This constant activity leaves the area congested, making it difficult for the road to function normally.

The diagnosis of CRS requires not only the signs and symptoms previously mentioned but also evidence of chronic inflammation in the sinuses. While an otolaryngologist may be able to use a special scope to see the inflammation and/or nasal polyps directly, imaging studies may be required to get a better understanding of the underlying disease. The most common imaging study used is computed tomography (CT) of the sinuses without contrast dye, which does a good job at detecting obstruction of the sinus ostia and other signs of chronic inflammation. Magnetic resonance imaging (MRI) is preferred if there is concern that the underlying disease extends beyond the sinuses. However, there are some concerns that an MRI may overdiagnose CRS and is much more costly than a sinus CT. Some of the most common findings reported from a sinus CT that reveals CRS include the sinuses filled with inflammatory material, obstruction of the sinus ostia, and thickening of the lining of the sinus cavities.

Other tests may be needed for other issues associated with CRS. Most patients with CRS have overlapping allergic rhinitis, so an environmental allergy test may be helpful. While most patients with CRS do not have an underlying immunodeficiency disease, additional immune system testing may be considered if there are recurrent episodes of bacterial sinusitis or when the symptoms of CRS are associated with other infections such as an ear infection (otitis media) and pneumonia. If there is an immune system problem, then it is most likely a problem with B cells producing antibodies, so the testing is generally focused on blood tests measuring for antibody classes and antibodies made in response to routine vaccines. Children who have nasal polyps need to get a sweat chloride test because nasal polyps in children are usually CF until proven otherwise. A chest X-ray and additional blood tests may be needed to investigate other potential systemic diseases such as granulomatosis with polyangiitis or eosinophilic granulomatosis with polyangiitis. In some cases, imaging may show signs of inflammation related to a fungal infection, which is called allergic fungal sinusitis. A biopsy of tissue may be needed to establish the diagnosis.

What Is Aspirin-Exacerbated Respiratory Disease?

Emily struggled during most of her childhood with seasonal allergies. After college, she developed a stuffy nose that was constant, and pressure was building up under her eyes. Eventually, she lost her sense of smell. Over-the-counter medications were not providing her much relief. She initially delayed seeing a specialist because she did not think they could help her. However, she got very concerned when she noticed that she was wheezing whenever she went running outside. Her primary care doctor initially prescribed her an inhaler to take every day, which helped prevent most of the wheezing she was experiencing. She eventually was diagnosed with asthma. However, over the course of a couple of years, her symptoms became progressively worse. In twelve months, she developed two asthma attacks severe enough to seek emergency medical attention and get treated with systemic steroids.

One morning, she started having a severe headache, so she took an aspirin. Within an hour, Emily's symptoms took a frightening turn. Her nose and sinuses felt like they were burning, she developed difficulty breathing, and she felt tightness in her chest. Emily panicked and drove herself to the emergency room. By the time she got there, her symptoms had almost completely resolved on their own. She saw an ENT specialist, who found that she had nasal polyps.

Emily's story is a classic example of aspirin-exacerbated respiratory disease (AERD), which used to be known as Samter's Triad. Roughly 7 percent of adults who have asthma also have AERD. The underlying cause of AERD is not fully understood.[*] This disease includes asthma, CRS with nasal polyps, and reactions to aspirin or other nonsteroidal anti-inflammatory drugs (NSAIDs). Other examples of NSAIDs include ibuprofen (Nurofen, Motrin, Advil), naproxen (Naprosyn, Aleve), and ketorolac (Toradol, Acular). Paracetamol is not an NSAID. The reactions to NSAIDs usually start within thirty minutes to three hours of ingestion. Often, the first reaction to NSAIDs goes unnoticed because it looks a lot like symptoms of allergic rhinitis, including a stuffy nose, runny nose, mild swelling around the eyes, and red eyes. Subsequent reactions to NSAIDs are usually problems with breathing, wheezing cough, and chest tightness, which looks a lot like an asthma attack. A typical rescue inhaler containing salbutamol can help treat these respiratory symptoms. It is rare for people with AERD to have a fatal reaction to NSAIDs.

There are some other signs and symptoms of AERD worth mentioning. People with AERD often report having reactions to alcoholic beverages, such as stuffy nose, runny nose, wheezing, and shortness of breath. Some people with AERD may also report having chest pain that can occur without exercising, which has been associated with higher levels of white blood cells called eosinophils. Some patients may report having ear infections and hearing loss as well.

---

[*] There is evidence of abnormal metabolism of arachidonic acid, which is an important fatty acid for cell membranes. In AERD, there are elevated levels of an inflammatory substance called leukotrienes, which contributes to the severity of asthma, as well as reactions to NSAIDs. There is also less production of an anti-inflammatory molecule called prostaglandin E2.

The diagnosis of AERD is typically made when there is the presence of asthma, nasal polyps, and a reaction to NSAIDs that involves respiratory symptoms. It can be difficult to establish whether someone reacts to NSAIDs, because they may not have been taking NSAIDs for many years. A small number of patients may also be taking too small a dose of the NSAID to cause a reaction. Also, they may be on either omalizumab (Xolair) or dupilumab (Dupixent), which could possibly block the reaction or reduce symptoms so that they are not noticeable.

Acute Sinusitis—Management and Treatment Options

Let's get back to Steven for a moment. He had persistent symptoms for over two weeks that were indicative of sinusitis and presumed to be caused by bacteria. He was prescribed amoxicillin-clavulanate (Augmentin) because it is effective against most of the common bacteria that cause sinusitis. If the symptoms were milder or did not last as long, we may have considered waiting to use antibiotics.

Nasal saline, drops, spray, or an irrigation device may help reduce symptoms because it helps remove mucus and irritants from the nose. Any irrigation device should be prepared with either distilled, sterile, or previously boiled and cooled tap water to help prevent a severe infection. NSAIDs and paracetamol may be used for pain relief and fever as needed. Inhaling steam may help provide some short-term relief. Antihistamines and steroid nasal sprays are not likely to be helpful unless the person has underlying allergic rhinitis.

Sometimes, sinusitis may lead to inflammation near the Eustachian tube, which connects the middle ear to the throat. This may lead to an obstruction known as Eustachian tube dysfunction (ETD). While Steven did not experience ear symptoms, sinusitis can lead to difficulty equalizing ear pressure during altitude changes, which may appear as ear popping or snapping noises. There may be ear pain or pressure, or hearing loss or a distortion in hearing called tin-nitus. If this occurs, then a short course of oral decongestants such as pseudoephedrine (Sudafed) may be helpful. However, these should be used with caution if someone has high blood pressure, glaucoma, or cardiovascular disease. Chapter 18 will cover more about decon-gestant medications.

I generally do not like using oral steroids such as prednisone for treating sinusitis. While there can be some benefits because it may shorten the time for symptoms to improve, if you weigh the poten-tial risk for side effects against the benefits, I personally believe that the risks outweigh the benefits in most cases. Oral steroids may cause several side effects, including a rise in blood sugar, weight gain, skin thinning, upset stomach, changes in bone mineral den-sity, psychosis, memory loss, anxiety, depression, and insomnia, as well as growth impairment in children. Each case is unique, so it's important to discuss with your doctor whether using oral steroids to treat sinusitis is necessary for you.

Chronic Sinusitis—Management and Treatment Options

For CRS, saline sprays or irrigation is recommended regardless of whether nasal polyps are present. If someone has CRS and has not had sinus surgery, then an over-the-counter nasal spray containing a steroid, such as Flixonase and Flonase (fluticasone), Nasacort (tri-amcinolone), or Nasonex (mometasone), may be recommended. However, if these medications have not worked or sinus surgery was done previously, then the steroid medication may not be reaching the sinuses well. There are a few ways to improve the delivery of ste-roids to the sinuses. A couple of examples include using a steroid such as budesonide that is in a vial for a nebulizer and mixing it with saline water in a sinus rinse bottle and irrigating the nasal cavities with this mixture. Fluticasone is a steroid that, in the United States, also comes in a device called XHANCE that may deliver the medicine closer to the sinus cavities because it requires you to exhale into the device to push the medication further than a typical nasal spray device. Oral steroids and antibiotics may be considered as well.

If someone with CRS does not do well initially with medical treatments, then surgery may be an option. A common surgical procedure is called functional endoscopic sinus surgery (FESS), which involves removing tissues around the areas where sinuses drain to help reduce the chances of ostia becoming blocked. FESS also removes nasal polyps if they are present. However, FESS does not treat the underlying cause of inflammation, so medical management should be occurring at the same time to help prevent recurrence. Another procedure that may be used is balloon ostial dilation (BOD), which uses a tube containing a balloon that is inflated in the ostia to open this space. It does not remove tissue, nor does it treat the underlying inflammation. BOD cannot treat all the sinuses, so FESS may be needed as well in some cases. Roughly one in five people who have sinus surgery require another sinus surgery, but most of those people have nasal polyps.

There is a class of medications called biologics, which are lab-grown antibodies that are now approved for treating CRS with nasal polyps. The three that have been FDA-approved are dupilumab (Dupixent), mepolizumab (Nucala), and omalizumab (Xolair). These medications are usually considered for patients whose sinus disease is not well controlled despite having surgery, for those who decline surgery, and for those who have severe asthma. Chapter 17 will discuss these medications in more detail.

Sam had CRS with nasal polyps. His allergy skin testing was reactive to dust mites and pollen. He started daily nasal saline rinses, XHANCE nasal spray, and Singulair. Fortunately, his symptoms significantly improved, and his sense of smell improved. Sam was very happy that he was able to start tasting food again. Due to this regimen, he did not require surgery.

AERD—Management and Treatment Options

Treating AERD involves managing asthma, nasal polyps, and NSAID sensitivity. Chapter 11 is dedicated to treating asthma, so the only treatment I want to bring up now is a class of medications that modify the ability for a pro-inflammatory chemical called leukotrienes to work. Montelukast (Singulair) is a medication that blocks leukotrienes from working and is commonly used to treat asthma and allergic rhinitis. This medication will be discussed more in chapter 11. Zileuton (Zyflo) blocks an enzyme called 5-lipoxygenase, so this medication, which is approved in the United States, stops the production of leukotrienes. Keep in mind that it may also cause liver damage, so liver enzymes need to be monitored regularly while taking zileuton.

Sometimes, we do not fully understand why treatments work. An example of this is aspirin desensitization for treating AERD. This treatment involves taking small, incrementally higher doses of aspirin until an effective "maintenance dose" is attained and can be taken daily. If the daily maintenance dose is stopped, then the effects of the desensitization process typically wear off within one to five days. There is no internationally accepted standard protocol for aspirin desensitization. Improvements in respiratory symptoms, nasal polyps, and quality of life have been reported from multiple small, randomized controlled trials using these protocols. However, taking daily aspirin can increase the risk of developing severe gastrointestinal symptoms such as heartburn, abdominal pain, gas, bloating, constipation, and diarrhea. This therapy is not as popular now because biologic medications not only help treat nasal polyps but also treat severe asthma.

Emily developed AERD and her asthma symptoms became severe over the course of a couple of years. Despite trying nasal saline rinses, Singulair, XHANCE, oral antihistamines, and a high-dose corticosteroid inhaler, she felt that her asthma symptoms were poorly controlled, and she struggled to exercise. Because of her severe asthma, she was started on Dupixent, which significantly improved her symptoms within a few months. She avoids NSAIDs, but her overall quality of life has gotten much better.

TAKE-HOME POINTS

- Most cases of acute sinusitis are caused by a virus and do not need antibiotics for treatment.

- The color of nasal mucus does not indicate whether antibiotics are needed to treat sinusitis.

- A combination of medications and surgery may be needed to treat CRS (chronic rhinosinusitis). Surgery does not treat the underlying inflammation that occurs with CRS.

CHAPTER 7

Food Allergies

How can food, which helps sustain life, potentially end someone's life at the hands of their immune system?

A month before seeing me in clinic, the parents of a nine-month-old baby girl named Isabella were having a regular morning in their suburban Chicago home. For breakfast, they were feeding her a small amount of watered-down peanut butter. It wasn't the first time she had eaten peanut butter, and she had done well previously. Her parents had introduced peanut butter when she was six months old because their pediatrician recommended starting early. They had heard about rising rates of peanut allergies in the news and that introducing peanuts early may help prevent a peanut allergy. However, within a few minutes of trying peanut butter on that particular morning, the baby became fussy and inconsolable. Her entire body was quickly covered in hives. Her parents called their pediatrician, who recommended giving her Benadryl.

It wasn't working.

Panic set in when she started vomiting about fifteen minutes later, so they called 9-1-1 and she was rushed to the emergency room, where she was injected with epinephrine and given more medications. She was monitored at the emergency room for six hours and discharged home with a prescription for an EpiPen and instructions to her parents to see an allergist.

When they saw me in clinic, Isabella's family was visibly concerned. Her parents loved peanut butter and were trying to come to terms with the fact that their daughter might be allergic. They did not know anyone who had a food allergy, so this was all new for them. Her parents were scared for Isabella to try new foods and were looking for guidance.

Isabella's story is a classic example of what an allergic reaction to food looks like. If you have not seen such a reaction, then it can be hard to understand what it is like to live with food allergies or to have a child living with food allergies. This is especially difficult when the terminology is confusing and is often misrepresented in popular culture. I have seen many comedy sketches that go something like this:

Title:
I'll Eat It Anyway

INT. RESTAURANT—EVENING

A new age restaurant, the dinner rush is in full swing. The sounds of clinking silverware, jazzy music, and scattered conversations fill the air. At a small table in the corner sits Mary, a well-dressed businesswoman in her mid-thirties. Peter, a polite and attentive server, approaches with a notepad.

Peter (*smiling*)
Welcome! Can I get you anything to drink?

Mary (*politely*)
I'd like a Diet Coke, please. Also, I need to let you know that I'm allergic to dairy, so I can't have any dairy in my food, all right?

Peter (*nods, writing*)
Absolutely. No dairy. Period. Do you have any questions?

Mary
No, I think I know what I want. I would like the Pasta alla Norma without any cheese or butter.

Peter (*confident*)
I'll confirm with the kitchen to make sure there is no dairy, and I will be right back with your order!

TIME CUT TO:
A few minutes later, Peter returns with her dinner entrée. Parmesan cheese is clearly visible.

Peter (*sets the plate down*)
Here's your Pasta alla Norma, bon appétit!

Mary (*looking at the plate*)
Uh . . . wait a minute! Is that cheese?

Peter (*nervous*)
Uh-oh! You're right. I'm so sorry! I'll take that back and have the chef remake it right away.

Mary
That's okay, I'll just scrape it off.

Peter (*confused*)
Are you sure? You said you are allergic to dairy.

Mary (*shrugging, begins to eat the pasta*)
Well, it's not that bad. I'll be fine.

Peter (*watching Mary eat*)
I thought you were allergic.

Mary (*talking with her mouth full of pasta and cheese*)
Well, it's more of an intolerance at times . . .

FADE OUT

Does that scene sound familiar to you?

The term *food allergy* should not be a blanket term. There are many ways the body can react to food. When you think about someone like Isabella who reacts quickly to a food and needs epinephrine, that usually refers to an "IgE-mediated food allergy." This means that the immune system has created immunoglobulin E (IgE) antibodies that can latch on to a particular food, which leads to a cascade of events that can be potentially life-threatening when the immune system encounters the food again. Symptoms of a food allergy may consist of hives, swelling, vomiting, difficulty breathing, wheezing, passing out due to a drop in blood pressure, or a combination of these symptoms. There are many other types of reactions to foods that do not look like this nor are they caused by IgE, some examples of which we will go over. For the sake of decreasing confusion, whenever I refer to a *food allergy*, I am referring to an *IgE-mediated food allergy*.

Why Are Food Allergies More Common Today?

Let's get back to Isabella's story.

Like many other parents before them, Isabella's parents asked me, "Why did this happen? What did we do wrong?" Food allergies were completely new for them and no one else in their family was dealing with this.

Every time I hear that question, my heart sinks a little and I shrug my shoulders.

"We don't really know, but I can assure you that this is not your fault."

Like most chronic diseases, food allergy is most likely due to a combination of genetic and environmental factors. There is no singular cause for people to suddenly become allergic to food. There may be an evolutionary basis for food allergies. When an allergic reaction to food is severe, it is referred to as anaphylaxis. This reaction may have evolved to act as an overly protective mechanism against toxins encountered in the environment. However, the rates of reported food allergies have been on the rise in many developed countries. In the United States, the number of children with food allergies increased by 50 percent between 1997 and 2011 and increased by another 50 percent between 2007 and 2021.

When I was a kid, I had a cow's milk allergy that I eventually outgrew, but I knew only one other kid living with a food allergy. Now there are about two kids per classroom who have food allergies. This is not likely just because of better awareness of food allergies. There are many theories about why food allergies are more common today. For example, vitamin D is a nutrient that plays a major role not only in maintaining healthy bones but also in immune system function. Recent studies have shown an association between low vitamin D measured from blood samples and increased risk of food allergies in babies.

Another possibility involves the gut microbiome, which contains trillions of microorganisms that help with digestion and regulate our immune system. Medications used early in life such as antacids and antibiotics can potentially alter the diversity of microorganisms in the gut and have been associated with developing food allergies. This does not mean that babies should never get antacids or antibiotics, but we should not overuse these medications. The use of probiotics in preventing or treating food allergies is still under active investigation. I don't routinely recommend probiotics to my patients to prevent food allergies because we don't know what types of microorganisms and what dosing are required to help reduce the risk of developing food allergies.

The timing of introducing food to babies plays a role in developing food allergies. In 2000, the American Academy of Pediatrics (AAP) recommended that children at high risk for developing food allergies delay the introduction of certain foods: Delay cow's milk until age one year; eggs until two years; peanuts, tree nuts, and fish until three years. The AAP changed its recommendations in 2019 because there was no evidence that delaying the introduction of these foods would lower the risk of developing food allergies. The Learning Early About Peanut Allergy study published in 2015 was the first to show that early exposure to peanuts could prevent peanut allergy. Researchers randomly assigned babies who had severe eczema, egg allergy, or both to either start eating peanut-containing foods between four and eleven months old or delay introduction until they were five years old. Earlier introduction of peanuts reduced the risk of developing a peanut allergy by 81 percent. These children were followed for twelve years and there was still a 71 percent reduction in developing peanut allergies in the early-introduction group.

Introducing foods early does not completely eliminate the risk of developing food allergies. In fact, many adults are developing food allergies for the first time. One of the most common foods that adults become allergic to is shellfish. One of the reasons why shellfish allergies may have become more common is that shellfish are biologically like dust mites. They contain proteins called tropomyosin that have structures similar to dust mite proteins. Over time, the immune system gets confused and may react to shellfish because of these proteins.

Children with eczema are more likely to develop food allergies, and the rates of eczema have been increasing as well. If food encounters skin that has a disrupted skin barrier, then the immune system may think that food is a parasite and become sensitized to it.

Our environment may also be to blame. Global temperatures

and levels of greenhouse gases have been rising over several decades. At the same time, pollen counts have been higher and pollen seasons have been lasting longer than ever before. More people are becoming allergic to pollen due to the increased and prolonged exposure to it. This is important because the most common form of an IgE-mediated food allergy is related to pollen allergy. This is called oral allergy syndrome, which affects about half of people who are allergic to pollen. Essentially, the immune system gets confused when someone eats fresh fruits, vegetables, and nuts because the proteins found in these foods are like pollen. The most common symptoms include itching, tingling, and mild redness and swelling of the lips, mouth, and throat. Rarely, this disease can cause more severe reactions such as anaphylaxis. If the culprit food is cooked, canned, processed, and possibly frozen, then the symptoms may not occur because the proteins may be sufficiently broken down.

Food Allergy Testing

After Isabella's parents told me her story, I performed a skin test. Within five minutes of placing the test, the area where a peanut extract was placed on her back grew into a welt the size of a quarter, which confirmed that she had a peanut allergy. Her parents asked me whether other foods should be tested. I cautioned them against testing other foods.

Food allergy testing has a high false-positive rate, meaning that the tests, whether by skin or blood, may say you are allergic to a food when you're not actually allergic. During my fellowship training, I was taught that "sensitization does not equal allergy." Food allergy skin and blood testing are measuring for IgE antibodies that can specifically latch on to a food, so a positive test means that a person is "sensitized" to the food. Remember, symptoms of a food allergy may consist of hives, swelling, vomiting, difficulty breathing, wheezing, passing out, or a combination of these symptoms. If someone consumes food and develops these symptoms within a few minutes to a few hours after ingestion and this occurs on multiple occasions, then a positive food allergy test confirms that there is a food allergy. People can have a positive food allergy test and not react for many reasons. One potential reason is that the food may be broken down by the digestive system before the immune system has time to react. When many foods are tested at once as part of a panel, up to half of the tests that are positive are not truly positive. I often tell a cautionary tale to parents about food allergy panel testing.

There was a six-year-old boy named Jacob who had had eczema since he was an infant, and he developed hives after eating a dish containing eggs when he was three years old. At that time, a food allergy blood test panel was sent by his pediatrician, which showed that he was positive not only to eggs but to peanuts as well. Jacob's parents were told to stop feeding him anything that contained peanuts. He loved eating peanut butter out of the jar, though! To truly know whether he was allergic to peanuts, he went through an oral food challenge, in which he would eat small, incremental amounts of peanut butter in the clinic under medical supervision.

Unfortunately, within five minutes after eating a pea-size amount of peanut butter, he started feeling itchy all over his body. His skin turned red, and he vomited. After vomiting, he was quickly injected with epinephrine because he had symptoms involving more than one organ system. He did not vomit again, and his skin turned to normal color within about fifteen minutes. This is an example of how unnecessarily avoiding food may have caused him to lose tolerance to peanuts and ultimately become allergic. I don't know how common this phenomenon is, but it forever changed how I practice medicine.

The Challenges of Living with Food Allergies

Living with food allergies can be rather challenging. Imagine having to read every food label carefully and alert everyone that you have a food allergy. If the food touches the surface of a plate that is not properly cleaned, then a tiny amount of the food allergen may be ingested and may cause the person to be very sick. This is known as cross-contamination, which can be difficult to control. People living with food allergies are at an increased risk of developing anxiety disorders. In 2024, I interviewed Florida congressman Maxwell Frost at a TikTok livestream event about his experiences living with food allergies and his desire to cap the cost of epinephrine auto-injectors at the federal level. He told me about the psychological trauma that occurred after developing severe anaphylaxis from eating a pizza that he did not realize had almonds in the crust:

It did a number on me mentally. I developed an eating disorder. I would end up calling an ambulance six times in the course of just two months eating at restaurants or eating at home because I had these phantom pains . . . and there was nothing wrong, but it was that panic disorder. I lost a lot of weight in that year because I started skipping meals because I was scared to eat, and it wasn't until I took my mental health more seriously and went to a psychiatrist and a therapist and started getting ahold of it, and now I'm a lot better, but for about three or four years there I really dealt with eating problems in a very serious way. It was horrible for a year. I got better after that, but it really changed the course of my life. Now, I still randomly will have panic attacks when I eat.

Both the people living with food allergies and their families are more likely to be bullied. Public places such as restaurants, airplanes, and schools try to accommodate people living with food allergies. However, this can be at the expense of people who do not normally deal with food allergies and so may perceive food allergies as an inconvenience to them. Food allergy is a chronic disease that can be potentially life-threatening, not a lifestyle choice or a fad diet. Symptoms of a food allergic reaction can range from mild to life-threatening, and it is not possible by skin or blood testing alone to determine whether a future reaction will be severe. There are multiple risk factors for developing severe allergic reactions. Asthma is probably the most significant risk factor for death from food allergy anaphylaxis, especially if symptoms are not well controlled. This is likely due to the chronic inflammation that is present from asthma, which can worsen the ability to breathe during anaphylaxis. Delayed use of epinephrine increases the risk of developing severe anaphylaxis. Alcohol and exercise can worsen symptoms as well. A variety of medications have been implicated, including aspirin, nonsteroidal anti-inflammatory drugs such as ibuprofen, and opioids.

Food allergies are often not well understood. Many people confuse food allergy with food intolerance, which is a problem with digestion. Food intolerance usually causes gastrointestinal upset and requires significantly higher doses to cause symptoms compared to food allergy. There is also the term *food sensitivity* that gets floated around the internet and in casual conversations. Food sensitivity generally refers to any symptoms that are perceived to be attributable to food. However, this is a nonspecific term, and the underlying mechanism is not understood. There are many companies that sell food sensitivity blood tests directly to consumers, although the tests are not necessarily helpful for understanding which foods to avoid. They typically measure for a protein called immunoglobulin G (IgG). This antibody is produced by the immune system in response to the body being exposed to food. This type of immune response is a way for the body to tolerate food, *not* to become sensitive to it. I have seen many adult patients who hand me a stack of papers with the results from this type of test, and I almost always see a positive IgG level for coffee. That happens because a lot of people drink coffee! In these cases, a careful elimination diet may be helpful to determine what may be the cause.

There is a lot of confusion surrounding reactions to gluten, which is a protein found in grains such as wheat, barley, and rye. Celiac disease is not a food allergy. It is an autoimmune disease in which the abnormal immune response ends up attacking healthy tissue in your body, such as the small intestine. This disease can cause several symptoms, including abdominal pain, vomiting, weight loss, iron deficiency, dental enamel defects, arthritis, and a rash called dermatitis herpetiformis. A biopsy of the small intestine confirms the diagnosis. There are also people who have symptoms like those of celiac disease but show no laboratory evidence of celiac disease. This is nonceliac gluten sensitivity, also known as gluten intolerance. Wheat allergies are different because they can be potentially life-threatening. All these terms get thrown around as if they were interchangeable, but they are different problems with different treatment strategies. Either way, the underlying trigger should be completely avoided in any of these conditions.

Food Allergy Management and Treatment Options

I want to get back to Isabella's story. After her diagnosis was made, naturally her parents had a lot of questions for me. I will try to give as much information as possible about how to manage food allergies. The main way of treating food allergies is to avoid consumption of the culprit foods, and treating reactions if they occur. A written food allergy action plan can help people understand the signs and symptoms of a food allergic reaction. For milder symptoms such as a minor rash, hives, or an upset stomach, an oral antihistamine is appropriate. However, if anaphylaxis is suspected, then epinephrine is the first treatment and should be given quickly. I also introduced to Isabella's parents the concept of emerging treatments such as oral immunotherapy and omalizumab, which will be covered in subsequent chapters.

They asked me, "Should we avoid foods that say, 'May contain peanuts'?"

In the United States, all food labels are required by law to list the top nine major food allergens: milk, eggs, fish, shellfish, peanuts, tree nuts, soybeans, wheat, and sesame. If these food allergens are an ingredient in the food product, then it will be listed after the word *Contains*. However, food manufacturers may voluntarily add additional labels, known as precautionary allergen labeling, such as "may contain." Other examples include the following:

Made on shared equipment with . . .
Manufactured in a facility that processes . . .
May contain traces of . . .
Not suitable for . . . allergy sufferers
Due to methods used in manufacturing,
    this product occasionally contains . . .

These terms are not standardized or regulated by the government, which makes them very confusing and probably unhelpful. We can't accurately compare them because they are essentially made up. An international group of food safety experts, the Codex Alimentarius Commission, has recently discussed trying to standardize the terms globally. If we can determine the minimum eliciting doses to cause an allergic reaction for the most common food allergens internationally, then that would help improve the health and safety of people living with food allergies and also would help reduce the anxiety that comes with reading food labels.

One of the challenges is to understand the minimum amount of food protein needed to cause an allergic reaction. It turns out that many people living with a food allergy may be able to tolerate a very tiny amount of their food allergen. As an example, there was a study of almost 400 children with a peanut allergy who ate 1.5 mg of peanut protein, which is about one one-hundredth of a peanut kernel. Less than 5 percent of these kids reported objective symptoms, which were mild, and no anaphylaxis occurred. About half of the children in this study were already eating foods that had precautionary allergen labeling, and they had no symptoms. Based on studies like this example, not everyone living with food allergies must avoid food products with these kinds of labels. It requires a nuanced conversation with your allergist to figure out what may work best for you.

"Do you have any other questions for me?" I asked Isabella's parents.

"We probably will," replied her mother. "Are there any resources I can look into to learn more about food allergies?"

I try my best to convey as much information as possible to families when their children are diagnosed with a food allergy. However, there is only so much information that one can process, especially during a potentially traumatic time. Questions tend to arise quickly after leaving my office. In the written food allergy action plan that I give to parents, I list organizations that provide evidence-based information. Examples include the American College of Allergy, Asthma & Immunology; the American Academy of Allergy, Asthma & Immunology; the Food Allergy and Anaphylaxis Connection Team; and Food Allergy Research & Education.

Keep in mind that there is an entire chapter on anaphylaxis later in this book as well as chapters on emerging treatments such as oral immunotherapy and omalizumab, which I highly encourage you to read.

Types of Food Allergic Reactions You May Have Never Heard Of

Up to this point, I have focused primarily on IgE-mediated food allergies. However, several other types of adverse food reactions can occur that may not necessarily be life-threatening but can make someone very sick.

Imagine a ten-month-old baby boy is brought to the emergency department with a fever and refusing to feed. He appears lethargic and his belly is fully distended. He has a thorough workup for an infection, including collection of urine, blood, and spinal fluid, and it does not show any infection. He is admitted to the hospital for antibiotics for a presumed infection and is provided intravenous fluids and does not take anything by mouth for several days. He improves and is discharged home. However, two days later, he returns to the emergency room with similar symptoms and his parents report that he had severe vomiting and diarrhea. This time, he is fed extensively hydrolyzed formula in the hospital, which means that the cow's milk proteins are broken down. He recovers more quickly, and it becomes apparent that this infant has food protein-induced enterocolitis syndrome (FPIES). This type of food hypersensitivity is not due to IgE, but the exact mechanism is not fully understood. It causes severe vomiting within one to four hours of ingesting a culprit food, and diarrhea can follow the vomiting. The most common triggers are cow's milk and soy, followed by rice, oats, egg, seafood, and peanuts. While most people outgrow FPIES from cow's milk or soy by the age of three, those who develop FPIES to other foods are likely to have more persistent symptoms.

Food allergy testing will not pick up on what is going on with some people. Sometimes, we may need help from a gastroenterologist to perform biopsies of the gastrointestinal tract to figure out what is happening.

As an example, I saw a toddler named Hannah who was the youngest of three kids. Her older siblings were completely healthy, and food allergies didn't run in her family. However, when she was nine months old, she started vomiting almost every day. Her pediatrician was tracking her weight, and it was decreasing quickly. Prior to seeing me, she had food allergy testing that was positive for peanuts, tree nuts, wheat, seafood, and eggs. However, because of her poor growth, she was initially evaluated by a gastroenterologist. When a child has chronic vomiting or diarrhea as well as poor growth, you start to worry that significant inflammation is occurring in the gut. They got biopsies of her esophagus and small intestines, which found high levels of white blood cells called eosinophils. These cells were causing inflammation in her small intestine, which was making it harder for Hannah to absorb nutrients. Eosinophils should not be found in the gastrointestinal tract in large quantities, and it is not normal for these cells to be found in the esophagus. Food can be a trigger for making this type of inflammation worse. She was diagnosed with both eosinophilic gastroenteritis and an IgE-mediated food allergy. Her diet became severely limited, and her family had to work with a dietitian closely to be able to help her get enough nutrients to grow and thrive.

Whenever I see Hannah, I usually can't sleep well that night, because I play in my head whether I gave the best advice to her parents. She has a unique situation where there are multiple reasons why she must avoid several foods. Will she outgrow some of these food allergies? We have some good data regarding how often people may outgrow some specific IgE-mediated food allergens and what blood testing levels need to be met before feeling more than 50 percent confident that someone has outgrown a food allergy. Between 70 and 80 percent of cow's milk, egg, or wheat allergies are outgrown. However, allergies to foods such as peanuts, tree nuts, seafood, and sesame are much less likely to be outgrown. When it comes to any of the eosinophilic gastrointestinal diseases, we don't clearly understand their natural progression. Some people will have symptoms on a consistent basis while others may have symptoms on occasion. In Hannah's case, after over a year of eliminating many foods from her diet, she has slowly been able to safely add back to her diet about half of the foods that she was previously avoiding. It took multiple visits with her gastroenterologist for biopsies and with me for food allergy blood testing to come up with a plan for her. I hope that Hannah doesn't have a significant relapse of symptoms. Only time will tell. For now, she is thriving, and we are all thrilled.

A related condition called eosinophilic esophagitis (EOE) has become more common, and it can occur in both kids and adults.

When eosinophils are causing inflammation in the esophagus in younger kids, it can cause feeding problems, abdominal pain, and vomiting; in adults, it can cause difficulty swallowing (dysphagia), chest pain, heartburn, and food getting stuck in the esophagus (food impaction). Eosinophilic inflammation may be triggered by various foods, and the most common ones include cow's milk, wheat, and eggs. Elimination diets can be helpful in treating EOE. Allergists used to routinely perform food allergy skin testing to try to help with identifying an elimination diet. However, as we have learned more about the underlying mechanisms of EOE, it turns out that skin testing is not very helpful in guiding the discussion surrounding what foods to avoid. There are medications that can help treat EOE as well, including proton pump inhibitors normally used to treat gastroesophageal reflux disease, swallowing steroids to coat the esophagus, and the biologic medication dupilumab.

Ultimately, managing food allergies comes down to managing risk. One of my mentors in fellowship training, Dr. Leonard Bacharier, would tell his patients and their families an analogy that I have adapted to my clinical practice:

Imagine there are two families who need to travel from California to Illinois by plane. One family is so nervous about the idea that their plane could crash that they decide to have each family member fly on separate planes to get to Illinois so that if one plane crashes, the rest of the family can still survive. The other family flying to Illinois is extremely carefree and decide that they want to get there faster, so they decide to fly together and skydive off the plane without a parachute.

I know this analogy seems a bit extreme, but clearly one family is extremely nervous, and the other family is dangerously carefree. It is crucial for people living with food allergies and their families to find a balance between being vigilant and reducing the anxiety that comes from dealing with this chronic disease. Food allergies must be taken seriously because they can make people very sick. Fatal food allergic reactions are rare, but they are tragic and often are reported on national news and social media. However, most people living with food allergies can have a happy, healthy, and full life.

TAKE-HOME POINTS

- *Food allergies* is often used as a blanket term, but there are many ways the body can react to foods.

- A small amount of food allergen can potentially provoke an allergic reaction, but precautionary allergen labels may be meaningless for many people.

- Avoiding the culprit food and treating accidental reactions are the mainstay of treatment.

- Finding a balance in the level of vigilance surrounding food avoidance is crucial for maintaining a healthy lifestyle.

CHAPTER 8

Eczema

Eric was an energetic three-year-old who was always on the move. He never seemed to stop moving and always kept his parents on their toes. He also had severe eczema and never stopped scratching his skin. Almost his entire body was covered in patches of a dry, red rash with scratch marks. His lips and fingers were cracked, and his arms and legs occasionally had pus oozing from the rash. He had a hard time listening to anyone because he didn't sleep well and was constantly scratching himself. On most mornings, his parents would find that his sheets were covered in drops of blood and a lot of dry skin flakes. His skin got infected multiple times, which required several rounds of antibiotics.

His parents had tried everything—bathing him frequently, bathing less frequently, bleach baths, and various creams or ointments. They went to a dermatologist who prescribed some higher-strength steroid creams, but his skin would not get fully cleared. Eric's parents felt terrible that their son was feeling miserable. The entire household could not sleep, and it was taking a toll on them. They came to me for a second opinion on what else could be done.

What Is Eczema?

Eczema is a term used to describe chronic, itchy, inflammatory skin conditions. It is often referred to as atopic dermatitis, which is the most common type. In this chapter, I may use these terms interchangeably to help decrease confusion when I talk about other types of eczema. Most of the time, eczema starts before a child turns five, but it can start in adulthood as well.

Even though Eric's parents had been diligently trying to get his skin under control based on their doctor's recommendations, they admitted to me that they did not really understand what eczema is and what was going on with his skin. With every patient I see for eczema, I explain to them what we know about it and what potentially causes the skin to become worse. However, we are still learning about the underlying mechanisms of this disease. Exactly how eczema develops is not fully understood.

A family history of eczema, asthma, or allergic rhinitis is the strongest risk factor for developing eczema. Families may pass down genetic variants that can increase the risk of developing eczema. The most well-known genetic variant occurs in the *FLG* gene, which encodes for a protein called filaggrin. This protein helps maintain a healthy skin barrier. Think of filaggrin as the mortar between bricks in a wall. Just as mortar holds bricks tightly together to create a weatherproof structure, filaggrin proteins bind skin cells to create a strong barrier. If filaggrin proteins are not functional, then the skin barrier is disrupted, which promotes the skin's drying out and leads to eczema forming.

Eczema causes the skin to feel itchy, but why does this happen? There are multiple reasons. The bacteria on the skin are less diverse and contain more *Staphylococcus aureus* bacteria, which increases the risk of skin infections. These bacteria also secrete substances called proteases that promote itching, possibly to help move the bacteria around so that they have more room to thrive. There are other chemicals such as histamine and cytokines (e.g., IL-31) that promote itching.

The immune system in the skin functions differently in people living with eczema. It is often referred to as "type 2 inflammation" because of a specific type of T cell, Th2. These cells are activated by various substances called alarmins. Th2 cells release cytokines IL-4 and IL-13, which promote further inflammation and lead to B cells producing IgE antibodies. It is unclear whether this inflammation is triggered by the faulty skin barrier function or by the skewed immune response.

Why Is Eczema Becoming More Common?

Around 7 percent of Americans have eczema, but rates in other countries vary between 5 percent and over 20 percent. Eczema has become more common globally. A recent study collected data from fourteen countries and analyzed over 100,000 children and adolescents. They found that over the past twenty-seven years, there has been roughly a 1 percent increase in eczema prevalence every ten years.

The increase in eczema prevalence is more pronounced in urban areas. Air pollution, increased water hardness, and exposure to tobacco smoke appear to increase the risk of developing eczema. Children who live in rural areas are exposed to farm animals and their microorganisms, which may provide protection against developing eczema. One study in Norway suggests that seasonality and climate may play a role in the increase in eczema prevalence. In 2010, Norway had an extraordinarily cold year and there was a relative spike in the number of new eczema cases reported. There were more cases of eczema in the winter and spring. How climate affects eczema risk is not clear.

One environmental factor that needs to be investigated more is skin care practices. Many parents use moisturizers for their babies. There are multiple studies addressing whether regularly moisturizing infants helps prevent eczema development. Unfortunately, the results are conflicting. Some studies report benefit while others show no difference. The conflicting results may be due to the difference in moisturizers used for the studies. Using fragranced lotions and bathing with soap often may play a role in disrupting the skin barrier early in life. However, it is unclear how much this may contribute to increasing the risk of developing eczema.

Eczema may increase the risk of other problems developing. There is a growing body of evidence that attention deficit hyperactivity disorder, depression, anxiety, and learning disability are more common in children and adults who live with eczema compared to other people. This may stem from the debilitating itch that people with eczema experience, which can cause significant sleep loss. Let us think about Eric again for a moment. His parents found his sheets spotted with blood and dried skin. He was scratching himself regularly at night and not sleeping as much, which led to poor attention during the day. Older children and adults may have a tough time socializing because the rash can be hard to cover and becomes socially embarrassing.

When I was a child, I had eczema that affected my arms and legs. When I was in elementary school, the rash occasionally was on my face. I vividly remember kids asking me at school, "What happened to your face?! Did you get cooties?!" No, eczema is not contagious, but the teasing at the time felt like it was contagious. I was lucky that I could cover most of my eczema, but I could not tolerate wearing jeans because the material felt scratchy and made my itch worse, so I wore baggy cargo shorts or trousers for most of my childhood until my eczema resolved when I was a young adult.

Many studies suggest that most children with eczema will outgrow the disease eventually. A 2016 systematic review of 45 studies that included over 110,000 people with eczema found that roughly 80 percent of children outgrew eczema by eight years of age. However, some experts are skeptical of a resolution rate as high as 80 percent because many people who have eczema may see significant improvement as they get older, but the eczema may come back later in life.

What Are the Triggers of Eczema?

When I examined Eric, there was something I quickly noticed before looking at his skin closely: His clothing was very tight! Scratchy, rough, or tight-fitting clothing can aggravate the skin, leading to worsening eczema. Synthetic fabrics (e.g., acrylic, nylon, polyester) or wool clothing may aggravate eczema because they trap heat and may cause an allergic reaction. Soaps, detergents, fragrances, dryer sheets, and smoke are other examples of irritating substances that may worsen eczema.

Most of my patients with eczema tend to see me in the winter for their eczema flares because the air is considerably drier then. Low humidity promotes the skin's drying out, which makes eczema worse. Why? Because of the itch-scratch cycle. Dry skin promotes the itching sensation, which leads to scratching. While scratching temporarily relieves the itching, it damages skin cells. Substances are released in response to the tissue damage, leading to further inflammation and itching. The cycle continues, making the itching and rash worse.

While I was talking with Eric's parents, I noticed that he was trying to bite his hand. This may happen because the itching sensation occurs deeper in the palms of your hand. Scratching alone may not give temporary relief from itching. Biting, although not ideal because of the risk of infection, provides more pressure to help distract your nervous system and temporarily relieve the itching.

Hormonal fluctuations may worsen eczema. Stress and anxiety increase the release of the stress hormone cortisol. This can influence inflammation and worsen eczema. Sex hormones can regulate skin barrier function. Estrogen has a positive impact on the skin barrier, but progesterone and testosterone can negatively impact it.

Sex hormones can alter blood flow and change how much water is lost in the skin. This may lead to fluctuations in eczema severity during the menstrual cycle. Pregnancy may worsen eczema due to the significant hormonal shifts that occur.

Infections may worsen eczema. *Staphylococcus aureus* bacteria often cause skin infections, leading to an eczema flare. One of the most dangerous complications of eczema is eczema herpeticum, which is caused by a human herpes simplex virus infection. The infection causes a severe worsening of eczema, where the skin appears eroded, and painful or burning blisters are punched out in appearance and filled with clear or yellow fluid. This viral infection may lead to severe inflammation of the eye (keratoconjunctivitis), inflammation of the brain (meningoencephalitis), or inflammation of the liver (hepatitis). Before antiviral medications were available, up to 50 percent of people with eczema herpeticum died from these complications.

The role of environmental and food allergens will be discussed in the testing section of this chapter.

What Does Eczema Look Like?

If you have eczema, your skin is dry and feels very itchy. *Eczematous* is a term used to describe a rash that looks like a form of eczema. However, the appearance of eczema varies based on the person's age, ethnicity, and level of disease activity. The inflammation may appear dark brown or reddish purple if the skin is darkly pigmented, and pink or red if the skin is lighter. Over time, chronic scratching of the skin may lead to the skin becoming thicker and cracked. In babies and young children, the rash is usually located on the cheeks, scalp, and the skin over the outside of joints such as the elbows. The diaper area does not usually contain eczema, likely because it is consistently moist. In older kids and teenagers, the rash moves toward the skin of joints that bend in, such as the inner elbows (antecubital fossa) and the back of the knees (popliteal fossa). These are known as flexural surfaces. The wrists and ankles may be affected as well. Adults also experience flexural involvement, but they also have eczema on their face and neck. The hands, ankles, eyelids, and lips may be involved, regardless of the person's age.

Mara worked as a respiratory therapist at a local community hospital. She was constantly washing her hands to avoid getting herself or her patients sick. She worked long hours and there were always some tough moments throughout her work week, but she found her career very satisfying. One day, she had a particularly stressful shift, and she went straight to bed when she got home. The next morning when she woke up, her hands felt extremely itchy. This uncomfortable sensation sent shivers down her spine. Her hands were covered with tiny red bumps that looked like a little bit of fluid was inside each one. She called her general practitioner, who was not able to see her that day, so she went to urgent care. The doctor there prescribed a topical steroid. Mara was concerned because the doctor did not know what the rash was. After a few days of using the medicine as prescribed, her rash went away.

Her relief did not last long. The rash came back about one week later. Frustrated, Mara called her general practitioner again, and he referred her to me for further evaluation. When I looked at her hands, I knew right away that this looked like dyshidrotic eczema. Also known as pompholyx or dyshidrosis, this is a subtype of chronic hand eczema that can be very itchy and look like tiny fluid-filled blisters. The rash is usually found on the fingers but also may appear on the feet. I am not sure how common this condition is, but every time I post about dyshidrotic eczema, it tends to reach millions of people, and I receive thousands of comments from people who believe they have experienced this rash.

It appeared that Mara's trigger for dyshidrotic eczema was the emotional stress occurring at work. Metals found in jewelry, such as nickel, cobalt, or chromium, also may trigger a flare of dyshidrosis. Hands that are frequently wet or sweaty, as well as warm, humid weather or very dry air, can be problematic. Even smoking can make

114 · **All About Allergies**

this rash worse! However, in many instances, we may not be able to identify a trigger for dyshidrosis.

Another type of eczema is nummular eczema, also known as discoid eczema. This is a coin-shaped, eczematous rash that gets very itchy. It is often confused with ringworm (*tinea corporis*) because the two look similar. Over time, nummular eczema gets drier and scalier, and the rash may become lighter or less inflamed in its central part compared to the surrounding area. This rash has triggers similar to those seen with atopic dermatitis and dyshidrotic eczema.

Eczema Testing

Monica was the apple of her parents' eyes. She was nine months old when her parents brought her to my clinic. She was their first child, and they were very attentive. They took pictures of her every day, and they loved to sing to her and play with her. Their two-year-old dog was very protective of her. When she was three months old, her parents noticed patches of red, inflamed skin on her cheeks and arms. At first, they thought it was dry skin and applied a moisturizing cream twice a day. Her father had eczema as a child, so he had some experience in treating it. However, as time moved on, the rash spread across Monica's tiny body and appeared more irritated. Her parents took her to their pediatrician for help, and they were prescribed some topical steroids for suspected eczema. Her parents also tried countless moisturizing creams and ointments, and while her rash would get better, it kept coming back.

Her parents were desperate for answers. Monica's mother had heard on social media that food might be the problem, so they insisted that I do a food allergy panel.

"I need to get to the root cause of her rash," her mother told me.

I paused for a moment and gathered my thoughts. In this kind of situation, I understand that anyone would want to know what is happening beneath the surface. I spent additional time explaining the complex relationships between skin barrier dysfunction that may have been inherited, abnormal skin microbiome, and immune system dysregulation. We discussed various physical triggers for eczema. All these factors play a role in how eczema develops.

I acknowledged to Monica's parents that there are some observational studies and personal anecdotes that suggest food may cause an eczema flare. However, the more important question is whether eliminating a food will improve eczema overall. Recently, a systematic review and meta-analysis was published that examined ten separate randomized controlled trials investigating the risks and benefits of a food elimination diet for treating eczema. This study reported that there was only a low level of evidence that an elimination diet may slightly improve eczema in its severity, daytime itching, and sleeplessness. Also, it didn't matter whether the individuals in this study eliminated food based on food allergy testing versus selecting foods by trial and error. The benefits were minimal at best.

As mentioned in the previous chapter, eczema increases the risk of developing a food allergy that can be potentially life-threatening. A food elimination diet in a child with eczema may increase the risk of developing a food allergy. One study reported that children with eczema who eliminated peanuts from their diet until five years old have more than five times higher relative risk of developing a peanut allergy than those who did not eliminate peanuts. Also, there is a potential risk that elimination diets may lead to feeding problems, nutritional deficiencies, and poor growth. Children also have a higher risk of developing anxiety disorders if they have a food allergy.

After I explained the potential risks and benefits, Monica's parents weighed these options and decided to not pursue food allergy testing.

"Is there any other testing that could be done?" her mother asked.

I offered environmental allergy testing. Multiple studies have reported a correlation between exposure to aeroallergens, such as pet dander, dust mites, and pollen, with worsening eczema. Reducing exposure to these triggers can lead to an improvement in symptoms. Her parents agreed to get this testing done, and it turned out that Monica had positive tests for dog dander and dust mites! Besides reducing exposure to these allergens, what else could be done for her?

Eczema Management and Treatment Options

Before discussing medications, I spent a considerable amount of time with Monica's parents going over the role of a daily skin-care routine and minimizing potential triggers. The frequency of bathing is still up for debate. I personally believe that the bathing routine should be daily. However, soap should not be used on affected areas of the skin every day. Soap can irritate the skin and lead to skin drying out and worsened inflammation. Do not use a washcloth or loofah to scrub the skin, because it can lead to further irritation. A mild or soap-free cleanser is preferred. Skin care products should be fragrance-free. I prefer people taking a bath over a shower and spending roughly ten minutes bathing in lukewarm (not hot) water. Afterward, immediately pat the skin lightly with a towel, but leave the skin slightly damp. Place prescription topical medications on the skin first and then apply moisturizer all over the body. This bathing routine is often referred to as the "soak and seal" method.

Another way to help moisturize the skin, especially if there is an intense eczema flare, is to apply a wet wrap after bathing. This is usually done after bathing in the evening and after applying medication and moisturizers. You can use clean, cotton clothing if the rash is all over the body or cotton gloves or socks if it's a smaller affected area. The first layer of the wrap is moistened with warm water until it is slightly damp and then applied to the affected area. Next, a second layer of dry wrap is applied over the wet wrap. This wrap may be left on for several hours or overnight to help heal the skin.

For more severe cases of eczema such as those of Eric and Monica, a bleach bath may be recommended. If you have not heard of a bleach bath, it may sound scary. However, only a small amount of regular, unconcentrated bleach (5.25 percent sodium hypochlorite) is used to make a dilute bleach bath: 120 ml of bleach for a full-size standard tub (150 liters); 60 ml of bleach for half a bathtub of water (75 liters); or 2 tablespoons of bleach for a baby bathtub (15 liters). Soak for ten minutes and then rinse off completely with warm tap water. Potential side effects may include skin irritation and dryness, but these baths are usually well tolerated. Multiple studies have found that bleach baths provide a small benefit for those with moderate-to-severe eczema, and at low cost. It is unclear whether other bath additives, such as oatmeal, baking soda, salt, apple cider vinegar, and bath oils, provide significant benefits.

After I described a skin care routine, Monica's parents asked, "What skin care products do you recommend?"

There are both over-the-counter and prescription moisturizers available to help support a healthy skin barrier. However, the prescription moisturizers are often expensive and there is not a lot of evidence that they are vastly better than over-the-counter moisturizers. I do not recommend a specific brand of moisturizer because each person responds differently to these products. What is most important is to understand that it may take two to four weeks before you know whether a particular moisturizer and treatment plan works well, so buying a bunch of various products and switching every few days is not helpful. Also, the vehicle of the moisturizer, meaning how the product is formulated, can make a significant difference for some people. Lotions and gels have more water content and a thinner consistency, but they do not seal moisture as well as creams and ointments. When it is hot and humid, a lotion may be preferable, but during the dry, cold months, a cream or ointment should be used to help hold on to as much moisture as possible.

When there is a significant amount of inflammation, moisturizing may not be enough to heal the skin. There are various topical medicines that are available over the counter or can be prescribed by your doctor. I am not able to go over every medication available, but I can cover some of the classes of medications.

Topical steroids are the medications most used to treat eczema. They help reduce the release of various chemicals that promote inflammation. Examples include hydrocortisone, triamcinolone, mometasone, desonide, and clobetasol. The strength of the medication depends on its concentration and the steroid agent itself. For example, clobetasol propionate 0.05 percent is much stronger than hydrocortisone 2.5 percent.

While these medications are usually well tolerated, there are some potential side effects to be aware of. Long-term use of topical steroids may cause the skin to thin, appear lighter, erupt a new rash that looks like acne, or become allergic to the medication itself. Overusing high-potency steroids over large areas may lead to systemic absorption of steroids. That could lead to several problems, including osteoporosis and type 2 diabetes. Higher-potency steroids should not be used on sensitive areas of the body, because the skin is at higher risk for atrophy. If the eyes are exposed to steroids, then over time, it can lead to glaucoma or cataracts. There is also concern that frequent use of topical steroids can lead to topical steroid withdrawal, which is a condition in which the skin becomes red, burning, itchy, and inflamed. It often appears as significantly worsened eczema and can take weeks to months to improve as the skin barrier recovers. However, if you follow the guidance from your doctor and follow up with them regularly, these potential risks can be minimized.

There are several nonsteroidal topical medications that may be prescribed. Protopic (tacrolimus) and Elidel (pimecrolimus), called calcineurin inhibitors, do not cause skin atrophy or other problems that are caused by steroids. However, these medications can cause a temporary burning or stinging sensation when applied to the skin. In the United States there is also a black box warning from the FDA about a theoretical concern regarding a potential link between these medications and cancer. Multiple long-term studies have disproven this link, and warnings have been removed in Europe, the UK and Canada, but are still present in the United States, Australia and South Africa. Eucrisa (crisaborole) is a topical medication that inhibits a pro-inflammatory molecule called phosphodiesterase 4; it is FDA-approved for infants as young as three months, though it is not widely available outside of the US. This medication can also cause burning and stinging, but it is more common than calcineurin inhibitors.

Over the past few years, a newer class of medications has been released to treat eczema and it comes in both oral and topical preparations. These medications block the enzyme Janus kinase (JAK), which is involved in the inflammation that creates eczema. They may relieve eczema faster than other medications, but they can cause broader immune-system suppression. There was a large, randomized safety study of older patients who had multiple medical problems, including rheumatoid arthritis and cardiovascular disease, and were taking the JAK inhibitor tofacitinib. The study authors reported that people taking tofacitinib may have an increased risk of serious infections, heart attack, stroke, cancer, blood clots, and even death. The FDA put a black box warning on these medications to alert people to this potential risk. However, multiple meta-analyses, including dozens of clinical trials of JAK inhibitors for treating eczema, did not report these increased risks.

Eczema causes significant itching, and there are a number of therapies that can address this. In addition to some of the medications already mentioned, oral antihistamines are widely used, but there is not a lot of evidence that they are beneficial. Phototherapy using either narrowband ultraviolet B or A1 could help reduce inflammation and itching, but it can be difficult for people to access this therapy since it can be expensive, and few physicians provide it. Cyclosporine is an immunosuppressant medication rarely but sometimes used in the most severe situations for eczema in older kids and adults.

Eric had tried many different topical steroids and calcineurin inhibitors. His parents had a difficult time diligently keeping up with the skin care routine because he often refused to bathe. His skin was very tough to control, and his parents felt they had no other options. However, at the time Eric saw me, the FDA had recently expanded the age approval for the biologic medication Dupixent (dupilumab) to six months old. Dupixent is a targeted therapy that can help significantly reduce inflammation related to eczema. More details on this medication and related medications, Ebglyss (lebrikizumab) and Adbry/Adtralza (tralokinumab), will be discussed in chapter 17. After weighing the potential risks and benefits of this injectable medication, Eric's parents felt that even though it was only recently approved for kids his age, they had nothing to lose. Insurance approved the medication very quickly and after one month on this medication, his skin dramatically improved. I saw him every four weeks for the first three months while he was on Dupixent, and I will never forget the happy tears that Eric's parents and I shared after seeing Eric smiling for the first time in clinic. His hands were not cracked, and his skin was already 75 percent better than when I first met him.

"I could hold his hand for the first time in months," his mother told me.

Everyone was able to sleep well at night once his eczema was controlled. He was a completely different child. Eric was focusing better and, overall, was much happier. While treating eczema can be very challenging, there are so many more treatment options available than when I was a child. Controlling eczema not only heals the body, it also heals the mind.

TAKE-HOME POINTS

- Eczema is a dry, itchy, inflammatory skin condition, and we do not fully understand the underlying mechanisms of this disease.

- A food elimination diet to treat eczema is not likely to provide significant improvement, and it can be harmful.

- The skin care routine needs to be optimized to help maintain a healthy skin barrier and reduce the chances of an eczema flare-up.

- There are many medications available to treat eczema that are highly individualized.

CHAPTER 9

Contact Dermatitis

As a young child, Erin struggled with sensitive skin. Rashes that were itchy and sometimes painful would appear out of nowhere all over her body. At night, she struggled falling asleep because she experienced horrible itching. Erin came from a military family who moved around the country and even spent some time in Italy. However, her family was just getting by financially, and it was hard for them to figure out what was wrong. Erin's mother tried to help as best as she could by switching the family to fragrance-free laundry detergent and limiting Erin to gentle soaps, but her skin broke out in unpredictable patterns. She hoped that one day Erin would outgrow her condition.

For a while, as she grew older, Erin's symptoms seemed to ease. She could tolerate a few products to which her skin would not react as fiercely as it once had. However, when she was sixteen years old, everything changed. Erin's rashes became more severe, and even her usual body wash caused a stinging skin rash with every use. Hot water would leave her skin dry and irritated. There was also a peculiar rash in the shape of a circle just below her belly button. She developed other health problems as well, including hypermobility issues and intractable hiccups. She was desperate for answers.

What Is Contact Dermatitis?

Contact dermatitis is an inflammatory skin disease that occurs when the skin comes into direct or indirect contact with substances. This disease has multiple subtypes and multiple underlying mechanisms. There are roughly 85,000 human-made chemicals, and roughly 2,800 have been identified as contact allergens. One of the challenges with contact dermatitis is that it can look a lot like other skin diseases, such as eczema. If you suspect that you may have contact dermatitis, an allergist or dermatologist may be able to help you.

Contact dermatitis is usually divided into irritant contact dermatitis and allergic contact dermatitis. Irritant contact dermatitis, estimated to account for 80 percent of cases of contact dermatitis, is the result of direct tissue damage from irritating substances, as with a typical diaper rash. Allergic contact dermatitis is a delayed allergic reaction that can be caused by substances such as poison ivy and nickel. For allergic contact dermatitis to occur, an initial exposure must happen before the immune system becomes sensitized to the allergen. The allergic reaction occurs when there is a subsequent exposure, and it usually takes between twenty-four and forty-eight hours for symptoms to develop. It can be difficult to differentiate between irritant and allergic contact dermatitis, so for the remainder of the chapter, you will mostly see the term *contact dermatitis* to help decrease any potential confusion.

The rash usually appears red, itchy, and scaly and may have bumps. Sometimes, there may be blisters, swelling, burning, and warmth. The rash is usually located where the skin is in contact with the allergen, but the allergen can be transferred to another part of the body by touch. Common areas affected include the hands, scalp, face, and eyelids. There are some cases of contact dermatitis that occur only when the contact allergen is exposed to sunlight; this is often referred to as a photoallergic reaction. Examples include sunscreens containing benzophenones and fragrances, and various medications including griseofulvin, doxycycline, and sulfonamide antibiotics.

How Common Is Contact Dermatitis?

There are not a lot of studies that answer this question. However, one report that analyzed studies between 1966 and 2007 from some groups of people in North America and Europe estimated that between 12.5 percent and 40.5 percent of people have contact dermatitis. Other studies have estimated the prevalence to be around 20 percent. It is rare to see contact dermatitis in infants and young children, but the rates start to appear similar to adults' at around ten years old. The increased prevalence of contact dermatitis over time is likely due to prolonged and/or cumulative exposure to contact allergens.

A major risk factor for developing contact dermatitis is occupational exposure to contact allergens. The people most commonly affected include hairdressers, metalworkers, healthcare workers, construction workers, painters, cleaners, and people working in the food industry. Contact dermatitis is not required to be reported as an occupational disease in most countries (exceptions include those in the European Union, the UK and New Zealand), so the rates are likely underreported. Also, several skin diseases may be confused with contact dermatitis, such as eczema, psoriasis, rosacea, and fungal infections, so it may go undiagnosed for a while.

Erin became frustrated with how some of her friends, family members, and doctors treated her. Some people told her that her symptoms were "all in her head." Erin did not feel that she was taken seriously. Doctors initially thought that she had eczema, but Erin sensed that more was going on because her rashes did not look like typical eczema. She started looking into what could be making her rashes worse.

What Are Common Triggers
for Contact Dermatitis?

There are too many potential contact allergens to go over, so I had to find a way to create a short list that would be most helpful. The American Contact Dermatitis Society created the Allergen of the Year award to help raise awareness of substances that cause significant contact dermatitis as well as those that are not as prevalent. I will go through some of these contact allergens on which the award has been bestowed since the year 2000.

Nickel is the most common contact allergen in the United States and common throughout the world. In 1994, the European Union (EU) restricted nickel use in consumer products through the EU Nickel Directive, which helped lower the rates of nickel allergy, though it has not been eliminated. Nickel is commonly found in jewelry, zippers, safety pins, belt buckles, spectacle frames, mobile phones, earbuds, multivitamins, and coins. Nickel was named the society's Allergen of the Year in 2008. Erin's story is indicative of a possible nickel allergy because of the location of the rash, which was just under the belly button. It turned out that she wore several pairs of trousers that had buttons and belt buckles containing nickel, which she started to avoid. This helped reduce the chances of her symptoms returning.

Nickel is found in various foods such as oatmeal, beans, chocolate, and nuts. When these foods are cooked at high temperatures, nickel can be released. A food allergy to nickel is often referred to as systemic contact dermatitis (SCD) when there is a rash scattered throughout the body that occurs without known contact with other allergens. The problem is that a nickel-free diet is impossible since trace amounts are found in commonly eaten foods, and it is also very difficult to measure the nickel content in foods. Nickel makes up roughly 1.8 percent of the earth's composition, so it is seemingly everywhere. People who are iron-deficient may absorb more nickel from food since iron and nickel compete for absorption by the body. Eating foods rich in iron and vitamin C may help reduce the absorption of nickel. It is unclear how much a low-nickel diet helps treat SCD in this situation. However, if symptoms do not improve after four to six weeks of maintaining a low-nickel diet, then it is probably not helpful to continue.

Another metal to consider is cobalt, which is found in medical devices, tools, magnets, ceramics, cement, leather, and plastics. It was named Allergen of the Year in 2016. While cobalt allergy is less common than nickel, metals often contain both elements, so some people may be allergic to both metals. Although cobalt is found in many foods such as vegetables, spices, meat, dairy products, seafood, and eggs, SCD is rare for a cobalt allergy. There are a few case reports of allergic reactions to vitamin B$_{12}$ (cyanocobalamin), but this is exceedingly rare. I have never seen this. As with a low-nickel diet, it is unclear whether a low-cobalt diet helps reduce SCD.

Neomycin is a topical antibiotic that is often used to prevent or treat skin infections or wounds. It was named Allergen of the Year in 2010. In the United States, this antibiotic is found over the counter in products such as Neosporin. However, it is now recognized as a common contact allergen. As many as 13 percent of people in the late 1990s were allergic to neomycin, but the rate has now declined to roughly 7 percent. Now, healthcare professionals are moving away from recommending it for routine wound care. If you are allergic to neomycin, then you may become allergic to similar antibiotics, including gentamicin, streptomycin, tobramycin, and amikacin.

Several preservatives can cause contact dermatitis; I will talk in more depth about two of them. Formaldehyde is a preservative used in many products, including personal hygiene products, nail polish, wrinkle-free clothing, plastics, textiles, and protective gloves (its use in cosmetic products is prohibited in the UK and the European Union, and restricted in Australia and South Africa). It was named Allergen of the Year in 2015. Because of the potential sensitizing and cancer-causing effects, formaldehyde-releasing preservatives, which are substances that slowly release formaldehyde, were created to help reduce formaldehyde exposure. These substances include

DMDM hydantoin, bronopol, diazolidinyl urea, imidazolidinyl urea, and quaternium-15. They can be found in hand soaps, lotions, fabric softeners, shampoos, body washes, baby wipes, and mascara. On the other hand, parabens are preservatives found in medications, cosmetics, and food. Without these preservatives, the products would be contaminated with mold and bacteria. Parabens were named the Nonallergen of the Year in 2019 because they are one of the least allergenic preservatives available. However, there has been some controversy surrounding potential health risks and endocrine disruption with parabens. There are some studies that reported that parabens have effects on the body like estrogen, which may increase the risk of breast cancer. However, these studies were either in a petri dish or in mice and were not replicated in humans. There are several studies that support its safety and no definitive proof that parabens are harmful. The Food and Drug Administration (FDA) has classified parabens as generally safe (outside the United States, e.g. in the EU, the UK, South Africa and Australia, they are declared safe within strict concentration limits, with some types banned).

Fragrances come from both naturally derived and synthetic chemicals that enhance odors and were named the Allergen of the Year in 2007. These substances are incorporated into many food, cosmetic, and hygiene products. More than 2,800 fragrance ingredients exist and at least 100 are known allergens. Because so many different ingredients are fragrances, it is challenging to pinpoint what is causing problems. Essential oils have become popular, but they may contain high concentrations of fragrances that can lead to an allergy.

Erin noticed that whenever she spent time at one of her friends' houses, she would come home with a rash on her hands, neck, and face. Her eyes would get watery, and she would have headaches. At home, her laundry detergent was free and clear of fragrances, dyes, and masking agents, but at her friends' houses, they often used detergent that contained fragrances that she could smell. Over time, she felt less comfortable spending time in other peoples' homes because of the toll it took on her body.

Cocamidopropyl betaine (CAPB) is a synthetic detergent found in many products, such as soaps, cleansers, detergents, makeup removers, shampoos, contact lenses, and toothpaste. It was designated as Allergen of the Year in 2004. CAPB allergy usually causes a rash on the scalp, face, eyelids, or neck. Even though CAPB is milder on the skin than other surfactants such as sodium lauryl sulfate, it is more likely to cause contact dermatitis. If you are allergic to CAPB, there are several items you should look for in the ingredients list that are alternative names. Some examples include cocamidopropyl dimethyl glycine, 1-Propanaminium, cocoyl amide propylbetaine, and cocoamphocarboxypropionate.

Paraphenylenediamine (PPD) is commonly found in hair dye, furs, and henna. It was named Allergen of the Year in 2006. When PPD is used as a hair dye, it is allergenic before it is oxidized, so it is not problematic after the hair dying process is completed. The rash associated with an allergic reaction to PPD often involves the hairline, eyelids, and neck. While red henna is not very allergenic, when PPD is added to red henna to make black henna, then it has a much higher risk of causing contact dermatitis. PPD also goes by several names on ingredient labels, including 1,4-Benzenediamine, 4-aminoaniline, and PPDA.

Erin also noticed that several sunscreens caused her to have a rash. One of the common ingredients found in sunscreens that may cause an allergic reaction is benzophenone. This chemical was named Allergen of the Year in 2014. It was originally used as a preservative to prevent photodegradation in paints, plastics, and varnishes. Now benzophenones are found in moisturizers, hair sprays, perfumes, shampoos, nail polish, and sunscreens. It can protect against UVA and UVB radiation from sunlight. The most common benzophenone to cause an allergic reaction is oxybenzone.

Acrylate is a chemical compound that comes from acrylic acid. It is often used in paints, adhesives, and plastics because it helps material harden or stick better. Acrylates are also in products such as gel nail polish, eyelash glue, contact lenses, dental prostheses, hearing aids, bone cement, and floor polish. In 1974, methyl methacrylate (MMA) was banned by the FDA for use in all nail products because it causes contact dermatitis and damage to nails. There is still trace MMA found in some nail products, and there are other acrylates found in cosmetic products. In 2012, acrylates were named Allergen of the Year. Since then, there has been an increase in allergic reactions to acrylate to the point that, in 2018, the British Association of Dermatologists issued a warning that acrylates found in gel nails were causing many cases of contact dermatitis in the UK and Ireland. When the initial lockdown period started in March 2020 because of COVID-19, at-home gel nail polish kits became popular. The problem with these kits is that to properly cure the gel nails, a UV or LED lamp is needed to convert the acrylate monomer into the hardened polymer. If the nails are not properly cured, then the acrylate monomer can cause an allergic reaction. Symptoms of an acrylate allergy occur not only on the fingers, but frequently on the eyelids. Eyelids are sensitive to allergens, and they are frequently touched, so the allergen can easily spread there.

How Is Contact Dermatitis Diagnosed?

Diagnosing contact dermatitis can be tricky since other skin diseases may look similar. Allergic contact dermatitis and irritant contact dermatitis have similar features, but there is also eczema, dyshidrotic eczema, psoriasis, and seborrheic dermatitis to consider. Eczema and dyshidrotic eczema are covered in chapter 8. Seborrheic dermatitis is a skin disease that includes greasy, scaly plaques mainly on the scalp, face, eyebrows, and eyelids. There is not usually a significant amount of swelling or blisters, which can be seen with contact dermatitis. Psoriasis has the potential to look like contact dermatitis if the rash is confined to the hands and feet, but often it is found on the elbows and knees along with little dimples in the nails (i.e., nail pitting).

If there is concern for contact dermatitis, a lot of information needs to be gathered to help determine the underlying cause. It feels like detective work. This includes the time course of the rash, its relationship with work, hobbies, and hygiene routines, and the treatments that have been tried. If the rash improves while the patient is on vacation, then exposure at work may be suspected. Material safety data sheets may be scrutinized when gathering information. Seasonal variation in the rash could be a clue for a substance reacting when exposed to sunlight.

When contact dermatitis is suspected, then patch testing may be done, which some dermatologists or allergists may offer. Not every specialist does patch testing, due to constraints on time, resources, and training, so make sure you check before making an appointment to see a doctor. In addition, for those who have to pay, out-of-pocket costs can be hundreds of dollars even with insurance, and it may require taking off work multiple times in a week to get the test done.

A patch test is done by placing various potential contact allergens on the skin and covering it with a patch, which stays on for several days to see if a rash occurs. It usually requires at least three clinic visits during one week. The patch is usually placed on the back. During testing, people should avoid showering, exercising, and extremes of heat and humidity so that the test can be as accurate as possible. The test can be itchy and uncomfortable. While skin prick testing requires avoiding antihistamine medications, they can still be taken during a patch test. However, topical steroids and other immunosuppressant medications may interfere with patch testing, so some of these medications may need to be stopped prior to the test. Tanning may also interfere with testing because ultraviolet radiation may reduce the number of immune cells at the skin's surface, so tanning should be avoided for at least two weeks prior to testing.

There are several allergens that can be tested using a patch test. The thin-layer rapid-use epicutaneous (T.R.U.E.) test includes thirty-five contact allergens. The T.R.U.E. test is widely used as a basic standard patch test. Depending on specific exposures or workplace conditions, additional testing may be required. When a patch test is placed, it is initially left for two days so that the allergens have time to penetrate the skin. After the patient returns to the clinic, the test result is read between fifteen and sixty minutes after the patches are removed, so that any redness from removing the patch can resolve. A second reading is done to help differentiate between an irritant reaction that fades away versus a true allergic reaction that is a persistent rash. This usually occurs on day four or five. If the second reading is delayed, then some reactions may be missed, such as fragrances. For some people, a third reading may occur on day six or seven, because there are some allergens that take longer to cause a positive test, such as neomycin, nickel, and steroids. Yes, you can be allergic to steroid medications that are meant to suppress the immune system.

What if the patch test is not accessible? There are some strategies that may help pinpoint the culprit allergen without using patch testing. The location of the rash can provide clues to the underlying problem. For example, if the neck is affected, this may be due to fragrances, acrylates in nail polish, and nickel or cobalt from jewelry. You could consider switching to fragrance-free products and avoiding costume jewelry and nail polish. If the belly button is affected, then it may be nickel from a belt buckle or metallic button. A trial of avoiding metal belt buckles and using clear nail polish on buttons may help. When doing a trial of avoiding potential contact allergens, it is important to do this for a couple of months before deciding whether it worked. Keep in mind that experimenting with switching products can become costly.

Erin had visited a dermatologist who offered her patch testing. However, her experience only deepened her frustration. Her skin was so sensitive that she reacted to the adhesive that was used to hold the patch in place, making it difficult to interpret the test. The test did confirm her sensitivity to nickel, but most of her triggers remained a mystery. Erin left her doctor with more questions than answers and became determined to manage her skin on her own terms.

How Is Contact Dermatitis Treated?

After identifying the offending substances, avoiding them is crucial for preventing symptoms from returning. However, this can be very challenging to accomplish. Your doctor may give you allergen information sheets to help you with avoidance strategies. There are also several websites you can use to help. The information can be found from companies that make patch testing, such as the American Contact Dermatitis Society (ACDS; www.contactderm.org), SmartPractice (www.truetest.com and www.allergeaze.com), Chemotechnique Diagnostics (www.chemotechnique.se), and Contact Dermatits Institute (www.contactdermatitisinstitute.com).

When it comes to avoiding substances that can be irritating, I have a very important point to make here. When you see a product that contains a label saying it is "hypoallergenic," it does not necessarily mean that it is safe to use. While the "hypoallergenic" label implies a lower risk of having a reaction, skin sensitivities vary from person to person. Many of these products still contain substances that can become contact allergens. In fact, one recent study reported that of the roughly 200 skin care products labeled as "hypoallergenic" tested in the study, 73 percent of them contained at least one contact allergen or related chemical. Also, some products carry the label "unscented" while others say "fragrance-free." The key difference is that *unscented* usually means that while there may be no odor emitted by the product, there may be additional chemicals added to neutralize or mask the odors of other ingredients. "Fragrance-free" on products means that neither fragrance nor masking scents are used in the product. ACDS has a Contact Allergen Management Program (CAMP) that can help identify alternative products that may be safe to use. Access to this program requires that your doctor is a member of ACDS. SkinSAFE (www.skinsafeproducts.com) is another potential resource for alternative products.

I want to touch specifically on some avoidance strategies for nickel, since it is the most common metal contact allergen. Some yellow- and white-gold jewelry and metal components of clothing contain nickel, which can maintain prolonged contact with the skin. Switch jewelry to nickel-free alternatives such as surgical-grade stainless steel. Nickel Guard or clear nail polish can be applied to buttons, which may help create a barrier that lasts for a couple of wash cycles. Duct tape may work as well. Some electronic devices such as mobile phones and laptops may need a protective cover.

Handwashing can irritate the skin over time if the handwashing is excessive or done too forcefully. If your skin is sensitive, then wash your hands with gentle soap for at least twenty seconds under lukewarm water. Hot water can irritate skin. Rinse well to prevent any soap residue. Pat dry your hands with a soft, clean towel or let your hands air-dry. Make sure your hands are left slightly damp so that when you use a moisturizer on them, it helps lock in the moisture. If you have a prescription topical medication, it should go on before the moisturizer. Protective gloves may help reduce or eliminate exposure of the hands to hazardous substances. Some people may need to reduce or avoid wearing jewelry, especially rings.

When there is a rash, topical medications may be needed. Usually, a prescription for a topical steroid or calcineurin inhibitor is needed to decrease the immune response. Stronger steroids are typically avoided on the face because of potential side effects, including an eruption of acne, additional hair growth, thinning of the skin, and pigment changes. If symptoms are severe, an oral steroid or other immunosuppressant medications may be prescribed.

There is a common misconception about treating contact dermatitis, which I will illustrate with another story. Mason was an energetic ten-year-old who loved going to summer camp every year. When he went to camp, he had a mild red rash on his cheeks and legs. He had recently been playing out in his backyard and there is poison ivy in the area. His mother thought he had a rash from the poison ivy, so she gave him some anti-itch cream and sent him to camp. A couple of days later, his face became very swollen. The camp nurse called Mason's mother and told her that she tried

Benadryl, but this did not help his rash. His father took him from camp to their pediatrician, who prescribed an oral steroid, and it cleared the rash. Poison ivy dermatitis is a delayed hypersensitivity reaction to an oily resin called urushiol. The rash is a form of contact dermatitis and can cause angioedema as well. While oral antihistamines can help with treating an itch, this medication will not likely help the rash to resolve more quickly. A topical or oral steroid may be needed instead.

As an adult, Erin learned to control her environment as much as possible. She works in human resources and initially had some struggles because she was exposed to fragrances from her coworkers that would not only irritate her sinuses but also her skin. When she was given the opportunity to work from home, she was excited for the chance to take more control of her work environment. Over time, she learned that she needed patience to meticulously discover each trigger. Breakouts still happen from time to time, but they are not nearly as frequent or severe as they used to be. She has a couple of prescription topical creams she uses when her rashes return. Erin has come to terms with the fact that she is living with a complex disease that defies simple solutions.

TAKE-HOME POINTS

- Contact dermatitis may be difficult to distinguish from other skin diseases such as eczema and psoriasis.

- A "hypoallergenic" label does not necessarily mean that the product is safe for everyone.

- Avoiding offending substances can be a challenge, since contact allergens are found in many products.

- Patch testing may help identify substances to avoid, but it can be costly and time consuming to obtain.

CHAPTER 10

Urticaria and Angioedema

rank was a bubbly three-year-old always looking to play and easily tiring out his parents. He was very healthy and never had an ear infection. However, a few weeks after his birthday, Frank looked off. His parents noticed that his cheeks were flushed, and he had low energy. His parents checked his temperature and found that he had a low-grade fever. They took him to the pediatrician, who recommended testing for COVID-19 despite his mild symptoms.

The next day, his results came back; he did have COVID-19. His parents were relieved that his symptoms remained mild, and he was able to sip some juice and rest. However, a few days later, some welts started appearing on his belly and back. He became fussy as he was scratching his entire body. They gave him Benadryl, which helped heal his rash, but they were worried about him and took him to their pediatrician the next day.

What Are Urticaria and Angioedema?

Urticaria is a fancy term for hives. It is also known as welts or wheals. The rash is raised, often itchy, red or pink bumps on the surface of the skin. It can be as small as a pinhead or larger than a dinner plate, and hives can be found anywhere on the body. There are immune cells near the surface of your skin, called mast cells and basophils, which release various chemicals such as histamine that cause nearby blood vessels to become leaky. This leads to the formation of a puffy bump, a wheal, and redness around the wheal, called a flare, due to enlarged blood vessels.

Angioedema literally means "blood vessel swelling." This is a process similar to urticaria, but the chemicals are released in deeper layers of skin, causing the area to become swollen. Common places for angioedema to occur include the face, lips, tongue, throat, abdomen, genitals, hands, and feet. It does not necessarily feel itchy, but if it is accompanied by urticaria, then itching is likely to occur.

What triggers this process? While we can find the underlying cause in many cases of urticaria, especially if it's new, there may be no specific cause identified. I know this can be hard for people to cope with, but sometimes people must live with uncertainty in their lives when it comes to their health. This isn't unique to hives. Whatever health challenges you are facing now, just remember that there is a lot that doctors know, but not everything about our health has been figured out. Fortunately, urticaria and angioedema can be very treatable despite not knowing the underlying cause.

To help ease my patients' minds, I often tell them that their hives are caused by "twitchy mast cells, but we don't always know why they're twitchy." I believe that understanding some of the basic immunology concepts behind how urticaria and angioedema develop can help people better understand what is going on with their bodies. I also hope that additional knowledge will help people avoid unnecessary testing.

Acute Urticaria

Hives that occur for less than six weeks are classified as acute urticaria. There are numerous causes of acute urticaria. The most common cause for children—and a potential cause for adults—is infections, whether it's from a virus, bacteria, or a parasite. SARS-CoV-2, the virus that causes COVID-19, commonly causes hives, and its vaccine is also associated with developing hives in rare cases. As the immune system is fighting off an infection, it may release histamine for a few weeks. While infections can be contagious, hives are not. For Frank, his hives were most likely caused by his recent COVID-19 infection. Most urticaria due to infections resolve within a few weeks, but in some cases, I have seen people develop hives for longer periods.

Some of the triggers for acute urticaria are caused by the immune system producing IgE antibodies that are specific to the allergen. Medications, foods, stinging and biting insects, blood products, latex, contact allergens (e.g., plants, animal saliva), and environmental allergens are some examples. There are also substances that can directly activate mast cells that lead to hives, including opioids, muscle relaxants, the antibiotic vancomycin, and radiocontrast dye used for imaging studies. Nonsteroidal anti-inflammatory drugs (NSAIDs) such as ibuprofen (Nurofen, Brufen, Motrin) and naproxen (Naprosyn, Aleve) may also cause mast cell activation.

There is a type of food poisoning that could also lead to urticaria and angioedema, called scombroid poisoning. It is usually caused by contaminated dark-meat fish such as tuna and mackerel. Other types of fish may cause it, including sardines, tilapia, trout, salmon, and mahi-mahi/dolphinfish. Contaminated Swiss cheese may also be a culprit. Scombroid poisoning occurs when these fish are not chilled or frozen properly. This leads to bacterial overgrowth and the conversion of histidine in these foods to histamine. For Swiss cheese, the contamination is found in the raw milk prior to processing. When these foods are consumed, the high levels of histamine may lead to severe urticaria and angioedema. However, it can often be confused with anaphylaxis. Fish allergy testing will be negative in these people, which helps point toward scombroid poisoning as the diagnosis.

There are several key questions that may help uncover the potential causes of urticaria and angioedema:

- Was there any chest tightness, difficulty breathing, throat tightness, nausea, vomiting, abdominal pain, dizziness, or lightheadedness that occurred along with the hives? This may be a sign that there was a more generalized allergic reaction.

- Is this the first time the hives occurred, or is there a pattern emerging?

- Did any weight loss, joint pain, joint swelling, bone pain, or unexplained fevers occur as well? These could be signs of a more significant systemic disease.

- What happened a few hours before the hives started?

- Were there any recent illnesses?

- Were there any new medications or supplements?

- Was there any recent travel? Any recent sexual encounters? These questions may uncover the possibility of an infection.

In today's smartphone age, pictures are truly worth a thousand words. Take photos on your smartphone of the rash so that your doctor can evaluate them. It may not actually be hives! Urticaria can be confused with other conditions such as insect bites, eczema, contact dermatitis, drug eruptions, reactions to plants (e.g., poison ivy), or a rash caused by a viral infection (i.e., viral exanthem). Hives tend to move around, and distinct urticarial lesions resolve within twenty-four hours. If the rash resembles hives and lingers for more than twenty-four hours, then it may be a condition called urticarial vasculitis. A skin biopsy may be necessary if this is a concern.

As its name implies, acute urticaria will resolve within six weeks. Despite an extensive evaluation, the cause may not be identified. I have seen several patients who have sporadic episodes of urticaria that are short-lived, but the evaluation is inconclusive.

Chronic Spontaneous Urticaria

Paula woke up one warm summer morning feeling itchy. When she looked in the mirror, her face was slightly swollen and there were large, raised red patches that resembled mosquito bites on her chest and back. Thinking it was a mild reaction to some food she had eaten the previous night, Paula did not feel too worried about it. She took some Benadryl, and her skin felt better by the time she had to go to work.

The hives never went away. Each day, they would return and were getting worse. It felt like her skin had a mind of its own. Her hives would appear unpredictably. Paula could feel a tingling sensation initially, and then the hives would appear. This could happen pretty much anywhere—at work, at the gym, or at dinner with friends. After one week, Paula dreaded being around people. She couldn't sleep at night because she felt so itchy and ended up missing days at work. On some mornings, she would look in the mirror and not be able to recognize herself because her face would be so puffy. Paula tried everything—cold compresses, lotions, antihistamines, changing her laundry detergent, changing her diet—but nothing seemed to help.

At one point, Paula was prescribed an oral steroid called prednisone from a doctor at an urgent care. She had never had this medication before, but she did not like the side effects she was experiencing. Paula had trouble sleeping and became very hungry and angry. At thirty-seven years old, she had acne emerge on her face. On the other hand, her hives got significantly better, but after she finished the prescription, her hives returned worse than before.

Days turned into weeks and weeks turned into months, but Paula was not seeing an end in sight. She saw an allergist who did a lot of skin and blood testing, but nothing came back conclusive. Paula was prescribed high doses of antihistamines, but she still had hives occurring almost every day.

What is going on with my body? Paula wondered.

Paula moved from Texas to Illinois for her husband's job, and she came to see me for further care. After reviewing her history and previous testing, I explained to her that she had chronic spontaneous urticaria (CSU).

CSU, which affects approximately 1 percent of people, is indicated when urticaria, angioedema, or both occur frequently for six weeks or more. Most people experience symptoms for two to five years, but it may take more time to resolve. There are multiple theories trying to explain CSU, but none of them fully establish the underlying cause. The autoimmune theory suggests that CSU is due to the production of antibodies or other factors that may increase the release of histamine from mast cells and basophils. When I was an allergy fellow, we performed a test called the autologous serum skin test, which is done by drawing blood from a patient and performing a skin test with the portion of their blood that contains antibodies, called the serum. Up to half of the people with CSU have a positive test. However, this test is not used widely anymore because it's not accurate and it doesn't effectively change the treatment plan.

Paula was surprised that I did not offer any additional testing. Apart from her rashes, she did not have any other concerning symptoms, and her previous allergist had done a lot of testing already. It is rare for an underlying cause to be found by routine testing if there are no other worrying symptoms. Sometimes, limited testing may be helpful. I usually check for thyroid function since there is an association between CSU and thyroid disease, but I rarely find an abnormal result. Testing for food allergies is not helpful for people living with CSU unless a specific food is known to cause symptoms within a few minutes to an hour or so after eating.

Pregnancy may impact the severity of CSU. In an international survey of almost three hundred pregnant individuals living with

CSU, over half of the respondents reported that their urticaria improved during their pregnancy, while close to 30 percent believed that their urticaria got worse. After birth, almost half of the respondents reported that their urticaria did not change compared to when they were pregnant. These changes in disease activity are likely due to the shifts in hormones, which can change mast cell activity.

Physical Urticaria

One day, Megan took a shower before going to bed, and as she was drying off afterward, she felt her entire body becoming itchy. She quickly noticed tiny red bumps on her back, chest, and arms. Panic set in because she had no idea what was going on. She showed her rash to her parents, and they realized she was developing hives that looked like small mosquito bites. Her parents quickly gave her Benadryl. Within an hour, her rash almost completely faded away and her itching stopped.

The next morning, she felt tired, but the hives were gone, and she was able to go to school. She was having a hard time adjusting to her classes in her sophomore year of high school, but today was much worse. She felt like she was crawling out of her skin. Megan was scared that her rash would come back, and people would notice her. She just wanted to remain hidden.

That night, she took another shower, and within ten minutes of finishing, her hives returned. Just like the previous night, she took Benadryl and was able to fall asleep. Megan became troubled by this pattern she noticed. Why was she getting hives when she showered? The following night, she decided not to shower, and she did not develop any hives. For several weeks, she noticed that her hives were getting worse when she bathed, and she was feeling increasingly anxious. She tried taking the antihistamine Allegra, but it was not helping. She was scared to bathe because the hives were becoming unbearable. Megan's parents took her to her pediatrician, and they referred her to me to evaluate her.

When I walked into her exam room, I quickly noticed a foul odor. Her parents were visibly distraught. She admitted that she hadn't bathed in over a week. After she told me her story, I decided to perform a simple test. Megan placed her arm in room temperature water for fifteen minutes. Within five minutes of removing her hand, there were small hives all over her arm!

"You most likely have aquagenic urticaria," I told Megan and her parents. "Essentially, you are allergic to water."

Roughly a hundred cases of aquagenic urticaria have been reported in the medical literature. Hives typically occur quickly after water touches skin, regardless of the water's temperature. However, the salinity may play a role for some people. Because this is a rare disease, we don't really know why it occurs. It can be a very debilitating disease. I initially prescribed high doses of Zyrtec (cetirizine) and Pepcid (famotidine) for her, but that did not help her significantly. I combed through the medical literature to see what other treatments have been tried for aquagenic urticaria, and I came across Xolair (omalizumab), which is a biologic (see chapter 17), as a potential option. I felt that we got lucky because insurance approved Xolair for her, and this medication worked amazingly well. Within four weeks, Megan was able to bathe freely and had minimal itching associated with her condition. While she was not able to completely wean off antihistamine medications, her improvements were substantial.

Aquagenic urticaria is considered a type of physical urticaria, meaning that the hives are caused by environmental stimuli such as cold, heat, exercise, vibration, and sunlight.

The most common physical urticaria occurs when direct pressure is applied to the skin such as scratching the skin. This is *dermographism*, which literally means "writing on the skin." You may have seen people scratch their name on their skin and welts appear within a few minutes in the shape of their name! Sometimes, the hives may appear even if the skin is not scratched. As many as 5 percent of people have dermographism, but most people do not experience itching with these hives. Treatment is generally not needed unless itching is involved.

Cholinergic urticaria is most likely the second most common physical urticaria. These hives have a characteristic appearance because the wheal is usually small, but the flare is very large. They are usually triggered when the body temperature is elevated such as during exercise or bathing in hot water. Strong emotions and psychological stress may trigger these hives as well.

I saw a patient named Charlie who was a very active young boy. He played sports and loved swimming. However, Chicago winters were not kind to him. Whenever he went outside when the temperature was below 60 degrees, he would feel itchy and develop hives on any skin that was not covered by warm clothing. Usually, his hives would go away, without medication, within half an hour after going inside and warming his body. In my clinic, I placed a bag of ice water on his arm for five minutes and hives appeared a couple of minutes after the bag was removed from his arm. Charlie had cold-induced urticaria.

What concerns me about cold-induced urticaria compared to other physical urticarias is that there is a potential risk for developing anaphylaxis. Prolonged exposure to the cold during activities such as swimming may increase this risk. As many as a third of people with cold-induced urticaria experience anaphylaxis. Since my clinical practice is in the Chicagoland area where it can get very cold for several months, I am generally more cautious and prescribe my patients an epinephrine auto-injector just in case someone develops difficulty breathing or swelling in their throat. Fortunately, roughly half of people with this condition find significant improvements in their symptoms within five to six years.

Treatment for Urticaria and Angioedema

For all the types of urticaria and angioedema just mentioned, the treatment strategy is similar. If there is a trigger identified, then reducing exposure may help reduce the risk of symptoms returning. In general, NSAIDs and opioids should be avoided since they can worsen hives. Psychological stress can be a potent activator of mast cells, leading to the development of urticaria and/or angioedema. Therefore, maintaining healthy coping strategies is necessary, especially for people living with CSU.

There are various antihistamine medications that are used to help reduce the amount of histamine acting on skin. The newer, second-generation antihistamines that block the H1 receptor include Zyrtec and Piriteze (cetirizine), Claritin (loratadine), Allegra and Telfast (fexofenadine), and Xyzal (levocetirizine). Your doctor may prescribe higher amounts of these medications than are available over the counter to help calm symptoms. If that doesn't work, then an H2 receptor blocker famotidine (Pepcid, Pepzan) is often used. While this medication is normally used to lower stomach acid, it is an antihistamine. If it is becoming extremely difficult to sleep, then first-generation antihistamines such as diphenhydramine, doxepin, or hydroxyzine may be used at night on an as-needed basis. When high doses of antihistamines are tried and are not successful after six weeks, then a biologic called Xolair (omalizumab) is often recommended. More specific details will be covered in the biologics chapter, but for now, I want to share a story.

Ayesha transferred to my clinic because it was closer to her home. She had severe CSU that was so bad, her previous allergist had prescribed her Xolair injections to be given every two weeks. Normally, this medication is given once every four weeks. Initially, she was doing well until she contracted COVID-19. Her hives quickly became out of control despite high doses of antihistamines and double the normal frequency of Xolair. Ayesha was desperate. She couldn't sleep well and was missing a lot of work, so she was given prednisone on multiple occasions, which helped reduce her hives. However, when her steroid burst was finished, her hives would return, often worse than before. She was really struggling to sleep at night and was given doxepin for some relief. However, she felt like a zombie throughout the day.

While I don't normally like doing this, we had to resort to trying an immunosuppressant medication. Ayesha tried CellCept (mycophenolate mofetil), which is an immunosuppressant medication normally used to help prevent organ transplants from being rejected by the recipient's immune system. This medication can cause an upset stomach and deplete white blood cells, so she had to have her blood counts checked every couple of months. Within a few months of increasing her CellCept dose, her hives and itching got under control, and her white blood cell counts never significantly dropped. She was slowly weaned off CellCept and needed Xolair only once every four weeks. But this took about twelve months to happen.

One of the challenges of managing CSU is knowing when to taper or stop medications. Unfortunately, there is no test available for accurately determining the right time to step down treatment. In my experience, urticaria and angioedema need to be completely controlled for at least three to six months before medications can be stepped down. When someone is ready to stop antihistamine medications, they should not stop them abruptly, because that could cause severe whole-body itching. Instead, the dose should be gradually lowered to help prevent this rebound itching phenomenon. I have seen some patients have their urticaria return after it fully resolved. It's unclear how commonly this occurs, but I have seen estimates that as high as 17 percent of people with CSU have symptoms return.

For Paula, her symptoms were still not controlled despite taking high doses of antihistamine medications. After a lengthy discussion, she started Xolair to help keep her hives under control. It took a couple of months for the medication to start working, but she found significant improvements in her symptoms. It is unclear when she will be able to stop this medication, but Paula is more hopeful now that she is rarely experiencing itching or hives.

Hereditary Angioedema

Amy was an ordinary twelve-year-old girl who loved being active and was often hiking on the weekends. One day, when she was out in the woods with her family, she felt a strange tingling sensation in her mouth. When she told her parents what was happening, her dad had a bad feeling that he knew what was going on. They quickly went back to their car and drove to the nearest emergency room. By that time, her lips were extremely swollen. She did not feel itchy or have any hives, but she felt very scared because she was starting to have some difficulty breathing. When the emergency room staff came to see her, her dad told them, "I am pretty sure I know what she has. I think it's hereditary angioedema because that is what I have."

Up to this point, I have talked about urticaria and angioedema that are due to histamine being released from the immune system. However, angioedema can occur for other reasons. Hereditary angioedema (HAE) is worth mentioning because it tends to run in families, and it can be potentially life-threatening. With HAE, there is an abnormal accumulation of a substance called bradykinin, which causes blood vessels to become leaky. That happens usually because a protein, the C1 inhibitor, is either made in low amounts or is dysfunctional. If the C1 inhibitor is normal, there may be other factors involved, such as coagulation factor XII, plasminogen, and kininogen 1. Swelling mainly occurs in the skin, upper respiratory tract, and gastrointestinal tract. An angioedema attack may cause severe abdominal pain, vomiting, diarrhea, and throat swelling that can be life-threatening.

While angioedema from allergic reactions normally responds to antihistamine medications and epinephrine, these treatments are not effective in treating HAE. Instead, the medications used to treat HAE focus on reducing the effects of bradykinin. Amy was lucky that she already had an established family history of HAE, and the hospital she was at had a C1 inhibitor called Berinert. Many hospitals do not keep HAE medications in stock because they are very expensive, and HAE is an uncommon disease. For example, Firazyr is a medication that blocks the bradykinin B2 receptor, but it costs over $10,000 for one dose and was at the time one of the top ten most expensive drugs in the United States. When I was in my allergy fellowship, I had a patient who needed a breathing tube because her throat was swollen so badly, and she needed three doses of Firazyr to reverse her swelling to save her life. When these newer medications are not available, fresh frozen plasma may be used, which is the liquid portion of whole blood.

For Amy, Berinert worked well, and she was able to get discharged home. Now there are multiple options for Amy to help prevent future HAE attacks. There are injectable C1 inhibitor replacements, as well as Takhzyro (lanadelumab) and Orladeyo (berotralstat). Once HAE starts, attacks will happen throughout Amy's life, but these therapies will most likely significantly reduce the number of attacks. Before effective therapies for HAE were available, roughly a third of people with it would die from suffocation. We have come a long way in helping people with HAE.

TAKE-HOME POINTS

- Additional symptoms outside of urticaria and angioedema may point toward a systemic disease.

- The underlying cause of urticaria and angioedema may not be found, but the rash is treatable.

- Long-term use of antihistamines is associated with developing severe itching if the medications are stopped abruptly.

- Hereditary angioedema is not treated with antihistamine medications or epinephrine.

CHAPTER 11

Asthma

One of the reasons I became an allergist was because of an experience I had as a pediatric resident. I was working in the pediatric ICU and there was a teenage boy named Carlos who was about to be transferred to the general pediatric inpatient unit. I did not take care of him for long, but I read through his medical chart, and it is something that I still carry with me.

Carlos had had asthma for most of his life and struggled to keep his condition under control. One day, his family took him to the emergency room because he was struggling to breathe. He looked very tired, pale, and was unable to speak in full sentences. His oxygen levels were dangerously low. If you listened to his lungs with a stethoscope, you would not have been able to hear any significant breath sounds. This is known as a "silent chest," which is life-threatening because air is not getting in or out of the lungs. After quickly trying to reverse his symptoms with various medications, it was clear that he was doing poorly, so he was sedated, and a breathing tube was placed.

The problem with using a breathing tube on someone who is having a severe asthma attack is that their airways are significantly narrowed due to inflammation and muscle spasms. This causes air to get trapped in the lungs, and the lungs become overexpanded. The process of intubation may trigger further narrowing of the airways, making it even harder for oxygen to get to vital organs. When a mechanical ventilator is used, the pressure from the air pumped from the machine may also cause direct damage to the lungs. However, in Carlos's case, he could have died from respiratory failure if he was not intubated.

While this boy fortunately survived, he developed severe complications from the asthma attack. He ended up having a stroke that left him paralyzed. His life will never be the same. I have not been the same since I met him. He was, by all accounts, a nice kid who was very outgoing and had a zest for life. I don't know the circumstances that led to his severe asthma attack, but I couldn't stop wondering, Was his asthma attack preventable? Over 27 million Americans have asthma, and roughly ten Americans die from an asthma attack each day.

Carlos's story motivated me to pursue a specialty that would help prevent people from having to go to the hospital due to an asthma attack. I didn't want to see this happen to anyone ever again.

What Is Asthma?

When I was in medical school, I learned how to present patients to a medical team, which is a crucial skill in healthcare. You must communicate effectively every major detail to others on the medical team to make sure that everyone is on the same page. It takes a lot of time and practice to communicate complicated and detailed information well. When a medical team is seeing their patient at a teaching hospital, a member of the medical team, such as a medical student or resident, typically presents the overnight events on the patient and their potential plan. This is often done in front of the patient. A lot of medical jargon is thrown around, and patients or their families may be confused by what is happening. These presentations seemed to benefit the medical team rather than the patient.

However, when I spent a few months in general pediatrics at the Cleveland Clinic, they had a very different approach from what I had previously seen. The medical staff was required to speak without any significant amount of medical jargon, and the patient presentations were geared toward the patient, not the medical team. At first, I had a hard time adjusting how I was communicating complex medical concepts, but I believe those skills helped me become a more effective communicator.

One morning, I saw a young boy named Alex who had been admitted the previous night with a severe asthma attack. He was living in an older house that was very dusty, with his parents and three siblings. His younger sister brought in a cold from day care a couple of days before and shared it with everyone else in her home, which caused Alex to have a harsh cough and wheezing. His rescue inhaler wasn't working well for him, so he was rushed to the emergency room and then admitted to the hospital for further care. After I finished presenting this information to the medical team and his parents, Alex asked me, "What is asthma?"

Up to this point, I did not have any experience explaining to a patient what asthma is. If you put ten doctors in a room and ask them how to define asthma, you will probably get ten different responses. This is because the symptoms of asthma—intermittent cough, wheezing, shortness of breath, chest tightness, or difficulty breathing—are not very specific and often have features that overlap with similar diseases. Various groups of experts have published statements defining asthma, but they are not consistent.

I felt embarrassed by my inability to give Alex a good answer, so I spent time looking into the literature for any creative ways to define asthma that most people could understand. I came across a paper from 2008 entitled "Children's Perceptions of Asthma: African American Children Use Metaphors to Make Sense of Asthma," which simply asked children to define asthma, and their responses were recorded. A twelve-year-old girl used a metaphor of a troll to describe her illness:

The troll is a little man in a green suit with big boots and a top hat. He is not very nice. He is small and sleeps all day in the dark, like under a bridge—kind of hidden, until I wake him up by the activities I do. When he wakes up, he climbs up the ladder to tell the air it has to pay to come into my chest. He says, "You can't go through until you pay. You need to pay." Sometimes the troll kidnaps your air.

I was amazed by her metaphor, and it made me realize that if you can describe what you are going through in your own terms, then you can be empowered to understand your health and make more informed choices. Whenever I am explaining medical concepts on social media or to my patients, I try to balance being as descriptive as possible with having as many people understand the concepts as possible.

Now I describe asthma to my patients as a chronic lung disease, meaning that the symptoms come and go throughout the year. The symptoms are not always the same, but they may include coughing, wheezing, shortness of breath, chest tightness, and/or difficulty breathing. The lungs have increased inflammation, which can lead to extra mucus production, plugging up the airways. The smooth muscles surrounding the lungs can be hypersensitive to various triggers and tighten the airways, also known as bronchospasm or bronchoconstriction. Triggers for asthma symptoms are usually known or identifiable. Examples include cold air, changes in weather, getting sick, exercise, environmental allergens, and laughing or crying. Asthma makes it harder for air to get out of the lungs, which is why it is classified as an obstructive airway disease. Wheezing is a high-pitched whistling sound that is heard from the chest when the airways are narrowed. Another way to think about this is to imagine blowing up a balloon. If you let all the air out by letting go of the balloon, then you will hear air rushing out of it. However, if you let the air out by slowing releasing your fingers but maintaining contact with the balloon, then the balloon has only a narrow point for air to escape. This is when you hear a high-pitched whistling noise that is like wheezing.

In medical school, I was taught that "wheezing does not mean that you have asthma, and you don't have to wheeze to have asthma." Wheezing is not required to have asthma! For some people, their only symptom is coughing. This is known as cough-variant asthma. Some people primarily have symptoms during exercise, so that is often called exercise-induced asthma.

Defining asthma can be especially difficult in young children. As an example, I saw Mark on a particularly quiet day in January. He was just eighteen months old. Most of my patients canceled that day because of the cold weather. However, Mark's parents really wanted to see me because he was recently discharged from the hospital. About one week earlier, he had developed a fever and cough that became worse at night. He was unable to fall asleep because he could not stop coughing. His parents became concerned because it looked like his chest was moving with more effort than usual with each breath, so they took him to urgent care. Mark was given a breathing treatment of salbutamol through a nebulizer, but his breathing was not improving, so he was transferred to the emergency room by ambulance. They did a nasal swab, which showed that he was infected with respiratory syncytial virus (RSV), which is a common cause of wheezing and breathing problems. From there, he ended up being admitted to the hospital for two days and receiving oxygen for a day. He was discharged home with a prescription for a nebulizer machine and some salbutamol breathing treatments.

Mark's parents told me that the pediatrician taking care of him in the hospital said he had reactive airway disease. This term is often used to describe wheezing in young kids when there isn't an asthma diagnosis. However, it is a nonspecific term that does not mean asthma. Almost half of children will have at least one episode of wheezing by the time they are six years old. Many of these kids don't end up having asthma, but they may carry the label of asthma. When the wheezing goes away, they may have thought they had "outgrown asthma," when they probably did not have it in the first place. If the wheezing starts during adolescence or later and the diagnosis is asthma, then most of those people will have asthma throughout their life.

How Is Asthma Diagnosed?

Diagnosing asthma can be tricky because there are several causes for wheezing and chronic coughing, and the underlying diagnosis varies depending on the person's age. In children, symptoms that resemble asthma may indicate an infection, a swallowed foreign body (e.g., coins, toys, popcorn kernels), cystic fibrosis, gastroesophageal reflux disease, or a structural abnormality. In teenagers and adults, there may be additional causes such as chronic sinusitis, heart disease, sarcoidosis, and panic disorder. Some medications may also cause chronic coughing. The classic example is a category of medications used to treat high blood pressure, called angiotensin converting enzyme (ACE) inhibitors. I don't want to give you an exhaustive list of potential causes because it would be overwhelming. However, I want to tell you a story about one of my patients to highlight a disease that mimics asthma.

Michelle had been a runner her entire life and was one of the best on her high school cross-country team. She was also a straight A student and was very attentive to her younger brother at home, who had cerebral palsy. However, over the past few months during autumn, Michelle's life drastically changed. Whenever she ran, she felt like she was suffocating. She was having a hard time getting air into her lungs and couldn't catch her breath. She felt terrified because it was happening almost every day. Her parents took her to her pediatrician, who quickly gave them an salbutamol rescue inhaler and said she had asthma. However, when she took the inhaler—whether it was before a run or for active symptoms—it didn't seem to work. Michelle and her coaches were frustrated that she was struggling, so she was referred to me to see whether she really had asthma or allergies. Sometimes, if someone is allergic to an environmental allergen such as pollen, this can trigger a hypersensitivity reaction in the lungs, leading to asthma symptoms.

I performed an environmental allergy skin test that came back positive for tree pollen, but her symptoms did not start during spring. It was odd that she had no relief from using her inhaler, so I ordered a pulmonary function test called a spirometry. In my clinic we have this small machine with which Michelle would inhale and exhale as much as possible through a tube connected to a computer. A clip was placed over her nose so that there was no air leakage. Some important data is measured by this test, including the following:

- Forced vital capacity (FVC)—the maximum volume of air that can be forcefully exhaled

- Forced expiratory volume in one second (FEV1)—the volume exhaled in the first second

- FEV1/FVC—the ratio of FEV1 to FVC, which is reported as a percentage

Michelle initially had three successful attempts at the test. Then she was given two puffs of the salbutamol inhaler and asked to repeat the test fifteen minutes later. The computer printed out her results, which showed a flow volume loop. This depicts the volume of air during her inhalation and exhalation. If she had asthma, she would have likely had a lower FEV1 and lower FEV1/FVC ratio, and the FEV1 would significantly improve after salbutamol was used. Michelle's test did not show any classic signs of asthma. However, her inspiratory loop looked a bit more flattened than what I was accustomed to seeing.

I suspected that something else was going on, but it was beyond my ability to confirm the diagnosis, so I referred her to one of my ENT colleagues. They used a special camera to look at her throat and found that her vocal cords were closing when they should have been open while she was breathing. This would explain why her inspiratory loop was flattened; she was having a hard time inhaling because her vocal cords were closing at an inappropriate time. Her findings were classic for a condition that goes by several names, including vocal cord dysfunction (VCD) and paradoxical vocal fold motion. Symptoms of VCD often look like asthma, but they do not respond well to typical asthma treatments. Typical triggers for VCD symptoms include exercise, emotional stress, and inhaled irritants such as cigarette smoke and cleaning chemicals. She was referred to a speech-language pathologist specializing in VCD who provided her with speech-behavioral therapy aimed at special breathing techniques to help regain control of her breathing. After several months of respiratory retraining, Michelle was able to play sports at a high level again.

This is an example of why it is important to follow up regularly with your doctors. If the treatment plan is not working well, then revisiting the diagnosis may lead to a new set of testing and treatment plans. Not everything is always what it seems.

Air Quality—A Hidden Asthma Trigger

Air quality is crucial for having healthy lungs. Every time you take a breath, your immune system in your lungs will decide how it will respond to foreign material. There are various small particles you breathe that can cause health problems. Small airborne particles are known as particulate matter, or PM. Examples of PM10 include mold, dust, and pollen, which are particles 10 micrometers (μ) or less in diameter. The smaller PM2.5 can be more dangerous; these include smoke, metals, soot, and combustion particles. These particles are tiny and can get into the smallest airways in your lungs. To put this into perspective, the average diameter of human hair is between 50 and 70 μ, and the average diameter of the tiniest air sacs, called alveoli, is about 200 μ. There are also various gases that are released from burning fuels and vehicle emissions, such as ozone, nitrogen dioxide, sulfur dioxide, carbon monoxide, and methane, that can be very irritating to our lungs. If you have asthma, then your lungs are especially sensitive to poor air quality.

During the summer of 2023, there was a significant amount of smoke that came from wildfires in Canada and spread through most of the continental United States. It was the worst wildfire season in North America ever recorded. I remember seeing a white haze like a fog all around me as I was driving to work on June 27. This was the wildfire smoke that had traveled from Canada. I checked the Air Quality Index (AQI), which is an essential yardstick from 0 to 500 that summarizes the level of pollution, and it was over 200, which meant the air quality was labeled "Very Unhealthy." On that day, Chicago had the worst air quality in the world. During the nineteen days when the AQI was over 100 and considered at least "Unhealthy for Sensitive Groups," there was a 17 percent increase in the number of emergency room visits due to asthma. I am not sure how many Americans died from the wildfire smoke, but I distinctly remember a news headline about twenty-six-year-old Destiny Mercado, who was the mother of two young children. She had severe asthma. During the peak of the wildfire smoke, she tried to stay indoors, but there were several cracks in their air conditioner, which did not filter out the smoke well. Initially, Destiny was rushed to the hospital and released a few days later, but her symptoms bounced back worse than before, and she was rushed to the hospital again. She fought as hard as she could and her doctors did everything they could to save her life, but she tragically passed away.

Air pollution may not be as obvious as wildfire smoke, car emissions, or smoking-tobacco products. There may be another significant source of pollution in your home—your gas cooker. There are more than 40 million homes in the United States that have gas cookers, and recent studies suggest that they are likely contributing to children developing asthma. When natural gas is burned at high temperatures, it produces nitrogen dioxide, which is a gas that can damage your lungs, increase inflammation in the airways, and reduce lung function. If you own a gas cooker and cannot switch to an electric cooker, then there are some options to reduce your potential risk of long-term exposure. Any time you cook, you should improve air ventilation by turning on the extractor fan, opening windows, and running an additional fan.

Asthma Management and Treatment Options

When I was a third-year medical student, I attended a lecture on asthma treatments from a pediatric pulmonologist while I was on a clinical rotation in general pediatrics. He showed us the asthma management guidelines from an expert panel, and there was a series of tables that gave recommendations for treatment based on the age of the patient and their level of asthma severity. The components of severity included the broad categories of the level of impairment and risk. *Impairment* was defined as how often symptoms occurred during the day, how often there were nighttime awakenings, how often a rescue inhaler was used, the level of interference with normal activities, and the degree of lung function impairment. *Risk* was defined as how many asthma attacks requiring oral or systemic steroids occurred in the past six to twelve months. *Asthma severity* is classified as being either intermittent or persistent, with different levels of persistent asthma (i.e., mild, moderate, and severe).

"Asthma is a cookie-cutter type disease," the pulmonologist told us. "The most severe category that you circle on this chart defines the level of asthma severity."

There are aspects of asthma management that do feel very cookie-cutter, with little variation. Once the level of asthma severity is defined, there is a set of medications that are generally recommended to prescribe. However, there are other aspects of care that go deeper. Asthma triggers should be identified so that exposure to those triggers can be reduced. As an example, if exercising in cold weather is a trigger, then shifting toward exercising indoors starting with a slow warm-up may be helpful. Allergy shots may also help with asthma in some individuals because they can help reduce allergic inflammation, leading to fewer hypersensitivity reactions in the lungs from asthma. More details on these strategies are covered in the allergic rhinitis and immunotherapy chapters.

One aspect of asthma management that has evolved rapidly over the past twenty years or so is the concept that asthma is not necessarily one disease. Asthma is likely an umbrella diagnosis for several diseases that have distinct underlying mechanisms. These diseases are called the endotypes of asthma. There are some tests that can be done to help identify which medications may be most effective. An entire class of asthma medications, called biologics, have become an important part of asthma treatment for people living with moderate-to-severe persistent asthma. Their effectiveness depends on the asthma endotype, which will be covered in more detail in the biologics chapter.

Most medications that treat asthma come in the form of inhalers or in a solution that is nebulized to create a fine mist to inhale. The two main types of asthma treatment either help prevent asthma symptoms or treat symptoms that occur. For people with intermittent symptoms, they may need only a rescue inhaler that contains salbutamol. This medication helps open the airways by relaxing the smooth muscles surrounding the lungs. In the United States, there is a newer type of rescue inhaler that contains both salbutamol and an inhaled steroid called budesonide that is known as Airsupra, and it can significantly reduce the risk of a severe asthma attack in adults. Doctors may instruct patients to use a rescue inhaler prior to exercise to help prevent symptoms. Many people who take salbutamol experience a faster heart rate because the underlying mechanism of salbutamol impacts not only the lungs but also the heart. Although it may seem counterintuitive to give a medication that may increase the heart rate shortly before exercising, this medication may help prevent asthma symptoms by helping to keep airways open.

People with persistent asthma generally must take medication every day to reduce the chances of developing severe asthma symptoms.

Most of these medications contain a small dose of corticosteroids to lower the level of inflammation in the lungs. There are significantly fewer side effects if the corticosteroids are inhaled compared to taken systemically, like by mouth or through injection. Higher doses of steroids are used when severe symptoms are seen in an asthma attack. My goal is to minimize the amount of systemic steroid used, because there can be several side effects that may develop with prolonged exposure to high doses. Some of the issues may include osteoporosis, muscle breakdown, bone damage, weight gain, diabetes, glaucoma, and increased risk of infections. Also, growth can be potentially suppressed in children. Inhaled corticosteroids may decrease their adult height slightly. One study of roughly a thousand children reported that their adult height was less than half an inch shorter if they were taking inhaled steroids daily for four to six years than that of other kids taking placebo medication.

Another medication that has gotten a lot of media attention recently also treats allergic rhinitis. Singulair, also known as montelukast, works by blocking the effects of leukotrienes, which are chemicals involved in airway inflammation. While this medication has been tolerated well by many people, there have been many reports of psychiatric problems linked to it. People have reported many symptoms, including increased anxiety, depression, sleep disturbances, nightmares, restlessness, and memory problems. The FDA has tallied over eighty suicides linked to this medication since 1998. Therefore, in 2020, the FDA put a black box warning on the package insert to alert people to these potential effects. If you are taking montelukast and are experiencing any mental health problems, please talk with your doctor about it.

Following Up with Asthma in the Clinic

I have to be honest with you. I am not a fan of medical TV shows. Part of the reason is because it's not relaxing for me. I don't want to watch aspects of my life on TV; it just doesn't provide an escape for me. Also, a lot of medical dramas are not medically accurate, so if I watch some of these shows, I may become obnoxious and correct everything I see. However, there is a scene in an episode of *House* that I can relate to and gives me a chuckle when I think about it. In season 5, episode 11 ("Joy to the World"), there is a brief scene where Dr. Gregory House is talking to a patient who has asthma, and he suspects that she is not using her inhaler correctly. When he asks her to show him how she uses her inhaler, she sprays it on her neck like perfume. While I have not seen someone spray an inhaler like perfume, I have seen some poor inhaler techniques. As an example, I once saw a child place an inhaler about a foot away from his face, click it, and then try to eat the mist that came out.

Many people do not use their asthma medications correctly, with estimates ranging as high as 50–90 percent. Some of the common mistakes I have seen in my clinic include not exhaling fully and away from the inhaler before taking the medication, not shaking the inhaler before each puff, not waiting for the recommended time before taking the next puff, breathing in too quickly, and exhaling too quickly. If an asthma medication is not taken correctly, it can increase the risk of developing an asthma attack. However, many people have reported that they were not provided with adequate asthma education or did not follow up regularly with their doctor.

People living with asthma should be following up with their doctor regularly and should be going over their inhaler technique during that clinic visit. Pharmacists can help with asthma education as well. A written asthma action plan can help guide people living with asthma about what medications should be taken when they are feeling well versus when they are experiencing asthma symptoms. I teach my patients the "Rule of Two" by asking them the following questions:

- Do you have asthma symptoms or use your rescue inhaler more than two times per week during the day or more than two nights in a month?

- Do you wake up at night due to asthma symptoms more than two times in a month?

- Do you refill your rescue inhaler more than two times in a year?

If any of the answers are yes, then the medications may need to change. Asthma is a chronic disease with symptoms not always present, but they can be severe. Always take your medications as prescribed by your doctor, but if you have any concerns, please speak with your doctor's office. Do not ignore your symptoms! Addressing the potential asthma triggers and taking the combination of medications that works for you will help you breathe easier.

TAKE-HOME POINTS

- Asthma is a chronic lung disease, and its symptoms can look like many other diseases.

- Air quality is crucial for maintaining good lung health, regardless of whether you have asthma.

- Understand how to take your asthma medications and seek help if your symptoms are becoming more frequent or severe.

CHAPTER 12

Anaphylaxis

O akley was eleven years old and he loved playing sports and being outside all the time. He was often seen laughing and playing with his twin sister, Olivia, and by all accounts he was kind and loved life. Most people did not know that he had asthma and was allergic to tree nuts.

In 2016, his family was on a Thanksgiving trip in Maine with their relatives. It was a cold day, and Oakley spent most of the time outside playing sports with his cousins. When he went inside, there was a coffee cake on the counter, and he took a bite out of it. However, his family did not know there was walnut extract in the cake. A few minutes later, he felt a little bit strange, and he noticed a hive on his lip. His parents gave him Benadryl, like most families would do, and his symptoms went away, so he went outside again to play for over an hour, not thinking much about his seemingly minor reaction.

When he went inside, he took a warm shower and got ready for bed, but things started to go in the wrong direction. Oakley started experiencing chest pain and vomited. He initially felt better and climbed into bed with his parents, but he vomited a second time and cried out, "Call 9-1-1! I don't want to die!" EMS arrived fifteen minutes later and gave him epinephrine, but it was already too late. His heart stopped and he needed CPR. He was rushed to the local hospital and put on a ventilator for four days. Unfortunately, he had lost oxygen supply to his brain and there was no activity left on a nuclear brain scan. The tough decision was made to stop the ventilator, and Oakley passed away.

On my social media platforms, I have shared Oakley's story many times. I have met his parents, who are wonderful people. His parents told me they had never heard of the word *anaphylaxis* prior to his death, and they wished they had had proper education on how to manage anaphylaxis at home. They started a nonprofit in his name, Red Sneakers for Oakley, to help educate others about food allergy and anaphylaxis. Oakley loved wearing red sneakers, so this organization encourages people to wear red sneakers on May 20, which is now International Red Sneakers Day, to help raise awareness about food allergies.

I shared this story not to try and scare you but to help raise awareness about how anaphylaxis can potentially be life-threatening, and I believe that everyone should understand what anaphylaxis looks like and how it should be treated. Just as with strokes and heart attacks, time to treatment is key to saving a life, and I am hopeful that you will feel more empowered to help someone if you are ever faced with a similar situation.

What Is Anaphylaxis?

Anaphylaxis is a severe, potentially life-threatening allergic reaction that occurs rapidly. Most symptoms occur quickly after exposure to an allergen. While some cases of anaphylaxis can resolve on their own, it can kill or disable you, so understanding the signs of anaphylaxis and treating quickly could help prevent severe complications. There are multiple ways the immune system could cause anaphylaxis. Regardless of the intricate pathways that may be involved, mast cells and basophils are activated and release several substances that lead to the symptoms of anaphylaxis. Histamine is the chemical that most people are familiar with, but several other chemicals are also released. Examples include prostaglandins, leukotrienes, platelet-activating factor, tryptase, heparin, bradykinin, and anaphylatoxins.

These chemicals travel throughout the body and have various effects. Flushing, itching, hives, and/or swelling of the skin may occur. The respiratory system may be affected, and a runny nose, sneezing, problems breathing, and/or wheezing may develop. In the digestive tract, nausea, vomiting, abdominal pain, and/or diarrhea may occur. These chemicals can also cause blood pressure to drop as blood vessels become leaky and move away from vital organs.

How Common Is Anaphylaxis?

We don't know how many people experience anaphylaxis, because there are challenges in diagnosing anaphylaxis and cases often go unreported. I have seen estimates that range from 0.05 to 2 percent of the general population will experience anaphylaxis at least once in their lifetime. However, I suspect that it is more common than we think. Roughly 500 to 1,000 Americans die from anaphylaxis each year. Delayed use of epinephrine is one of the most important reasons why someone dies from anaphylaxis. However, even if epinephrine is used quickly, there are very rare cases of death, so it is not universally effective. Regardless of how frequently anaphylaxis occurs, it is a worldwide problem that is becoming more common.

What Are the Triggers and Risk Factors for Anaphylaxis?

The list of potential triggers of anaphylaxis is enormous and it is impossible to list all of them, but we will go over some of the most common triggers as well as some of the more unusual ones. Essentially, if the substance is large enough to interact with your immune system, then there is a possibility that it could cause anaphylaxis. The most common triggers are foods, medications, stinging insects, and latex. This book has entire chapters dedicated to food (chapter 7) and medication (chapter 13) allergies. Here, we will provide more information about stinging insects and latex allergies.

Seth was an avid golfer who always found peace on the green. The sounds of nature and a perfectly hit golf ball calmed his mind. One fall afternoon, he was lining up his shot on the eighth hole when he felt a sudden sharp sting on his forearm that was very painful. He looked down at his arm and noticed that a wasp had stung him. At first, he thought it was a minor nuisance, but within a few minutes, Seth felt his throat tighten, and it became difficult to breathe. He knew something was wrong. He had a child with food allergies, so he luckily had an expired EpiPen with him, which he quickly gave himself. Within fifteen minutes, an ambulance arrived and took him to the emergency room. Fortunately, he was treated and recovered within a few hours.

Stinging insects, also known as Hymenoptera, include honeybees, bumblebees, hornets, wasps, and fire ants. Anaphylaxis that occurs from stinging insects is due to the proteins found in their venom and not the insect's body. Most reactions to bee stings happen just at the site of the sting, which is usually referred to as a local reaction. When the reaction is larger than 10 cm in diameter, it is called a large local reaction. When the symptoms happen in areas of the body away from the site of the sting, it is considered a systemic reaction. The distinction between local and systemic reactions is important because it helps predict the future risk of anaphylaxis if someone is stung again. A large local reaction does not usually require testing and treatment because the risk of a systemic reaction in the future is approximately 4 to 10 percent, and severe anaphylaxis occurs in less than 3 percent of stings. If you experience an anaphylactic reaction to an insect sting, then you need to see an allergist to get tested and consider treatment, because the risk of anaphylaxis is 30 to 60 percent if another sting occurs.

Most of the natural rubber latex produced comes from a sap-like fluid from the commercial rubber tree *Hevea brasiliensis*, which is grown in Southeast Asia and Africa. Latex is found in a variety of products. The latex-based products that have caused most of the cases of anaphylaxis include gloves, balloon-tipped catheters, condoms, adhesives from hair extensions, toy balloons, pacifiers, bottle nipples, and dental dams. While latex allergy is not very common nowadays (less than 1 percent of the population) because powdered latex gloves in hospitals are now avoided, there was an epidemic of cases in the mid- to late 1990s (3 to 9.5 percent of the general population) because of a significant increase in the use of these latex gloves. The increased use of the gloves was a response to the US Occupational Safety and Health Administration's issue of the Bloodborne Pathogens Standard, which required protective glove use. At that time, there was a limited supply of latex. To boost production, younger trees were treated with stimulants that increased the number of allergenic proteins in the latex. Also, the latex that was produced was not stored for an extended period, so there was less time for the allergenic proteins to break down during storage.

Currently, the people who are most likely to have a latex allergy are those who are exposed through their work. Examples include healthcare workers, first responders, food handlers, restaurant workers, hairdressers, construction workers, painters, gardeners, and security personnel. Children with spina bifida used to undergo multiple surgeries involving latex materials, so roughly half would develop a latex allergy until precautions were put in place. Between 30 and 50 percent of people allergic to latex are also allergic to some foods, a condition known as latex-fruit or latex-food syndrome. This is because the latex proteins are cross-reactive with proteins found in certain plant-derived foods such as bananas, avocados, chestnuts, kiwis, papayas, white potatoes, and tomatoes. When I see patients with latex allergy, I do not usually perform food allergy testing unless they have a history of reacting to a particular food.

Another important cause of anaphylaxis is radiocontrast media (aka contrast dyes) used for imaging studies. Many healthcare systems still have policies in place that support the myth that there is a relationship between an allergy to iodine-containing contrast dyes and a shellfish allergy. This myth started in the 1970s from a survey of patients who reported reactions to contrast dye. That study reported that 15 percent of patients who reacted to contrast media were allergic to shellfish. Since shellfish contains iodine, physicians and other healthcare professionals were taught that people allergic to shellfish were allergic to iodine, so they should avoid iodine-containing contrast dye. However, this observation was not fully tested. In fact, most people allergic to shellfish are allergic to a muscle protein called tropomyosin. Also, iodine is not an allergen. Our bodies have iodine, and it is too small for our immune system to recognize it as foreign. The reactions that occur with radiocontrast dyes are most likely caused not by the iodine alone but by other molecules present in the dyes.

Rosa is a nurse who spent years trying to uncover the mystery behind her unusual and persistent symptoms. She battled hives, swelling, and problems breathing in the middle of the night. After years of struggling with trying various allergy medications, she realized that her symptoms were worsened after eating meat. Her allergist tested her blood, which confirmed that she had alpha-gal syndrome (AGS). Alpha-gal is short for galactose-α-1,3-galactose, which is a sugar molecule found in most mammals except humans and some other primates. In the United States, AGS is associated with tick bites, mainly from the lone star tick, which is mostly found in the southern, eastern, and central states. Rosa had to avoid eating meat and learn how to meticulously avoid foods containing hidden animal products such as gelatin and vitamins. Many people also must avoid dairy products. AGS is becoming more common and may now be the tenth most common food allergy in the United States. It can cause anaphylaxis, but it is usually delayed up to several hours after exposure to alpha-gal. That is why many people like Rosa would wake up in the middle of the night with severe symptoms. If tick bites and the allergen are avoided, then some people may be able to outgrow AGS over time. Subsequent tick bites may cause AGS to become persistent.

There are several rare causes of anaphylaxis, including mast cell disorders (covered in chapter 14) and various physical triggers. People with cholinergic urticaria, cold-induced urticaria, and solar urticaria can experience anaphylaxis due to extreme heat, cold, or sunlight, respectively.

Some people are even allergic to exercise! This is referred to as exercise-induced anaphylaxis. If it occurs only in the setting of ingesting an allergenic food such as wheat, nuts, or shellfish and then exercising within a few hours, this is called food-dependent, exercise-induced anaphylaxis. It may happen because exercise can increase gut permeability to allergens. Alcohol and nonsteroidal anti-inflammatory drugs (e.g., ibuprofen, naproxen) may also worsen anaphylaxis through a mechanism similar to exercise.

Unfortunately, anaphylaxis can occur without an identifiable cause. A doctor can order a multitude of tests, and nothing turns out to be positive. This is referred to as spontaneous, or idiopathic, anaphylaxis, and may occur in up to two-thirds of adults who see an allergist for an evaluation of anaphylaxis. The situation is very frustrating and concerning because it is unclear to us how frequently anaphylaxis may occur without our knowing the underlying trigger.

There are several factors that may affect how commonly anaphylaxis occurs as well as its level of severity. Anaphylaxis tends to occur more frequently in areas with less sunlight, which means that vitamin D may play a role, but this hypothesis has not been thoroughly tested. Males under age fifteen and females over age fifteen are more likely affected, which implies that hormonal shifts influence anaphylaxis. The route of exposure to the provoking substance also plays a role. The faster the immune system sees the substance, the higher the chance that the substance will provoke anaphylaxis. As an example, a medication that is injected is more likely to cause anaphylaxis than when it is ingested. Poorly controlled asthma is a significant risk factor for severe anaphylaxis. There are several reasons why this may be the case. For example, poorly controlled asthma can lead to increased airway inflammation, which can worsen an anaphylactic reaction. Also, there may be a delayed response to epinephrine in treating anaphylaxis if asthma is poorly controlled.

How Is Anaphylaxis Diagnosed?

Anaphylaxis is usually a clinical diagnosis based on what has recently happened with the person and their symptoms. Diagnostic criteria created by a group of international experts are summarized here. Anaphylaxis is highly likely when any one of these three scenarios occurs:

1. An illness that happens within minutes to a few hours and includes involvement of the skin, such as hives, itching, flushing, and/or swollen lips-tongue-uvula AND either
    a. Respiratory problems such as wheezing or trouble breathing, or
    b. Reduced blood pressure that may appear as passing out or losing bowel or bladder function

2. Two or more of the following that occur quickly after exposure to a likely allergen, within minutes to a few hours:
    a. Skin: hives, itching, flushing, swollen lips-tongue-uvula
    b. Respiratory problems such as wheezing or problems breathing
    c. Reduced blood pressure that may appear as passing out or losing bowel or bladder function

    d. Persistent gastrointestinal problems such as vomiting, diarrhea, or crampy abdominal pain

3. Reduced blood pressure after exposure to a known allergen for that person

Sometimes, blood and urine tests may help diagnose anaphylaxis or rule out other conditions. Tryptase, a protein released from mast cells during anaphylaxis, can be measured in a blood test. Histamine released by the immune system breaks down quickly in the blood into substances such as N-methylhistamine that can be measured in the urine. Symptoms of anaphylaxis can be confused with several conditions, including an asthma attack, vasovagal syncope (fainting), vocal cord dysfunction, panic attacks, swallowing a foreign body (mostly in kids), and seizures.

In addition, some people may experience scombroid food poisoning, which happens because someone eats fresh, canned, or smoked fish that has high histamine levels due to improper processing or storage. The fish may taste normal, but it can cause very similar symptoms to anaphylaxis. People with scombroid food poisoning are often treated as if they have anaphylaxis, but when they are tested for food allergies later, their skin and blood tests are negative for seafood allergies.

You may have heard people use the terms *anaphylactic shock* and *anaphylaxis* interchangeably. However, they are not the same. Anaphylactic shock refers to when the process of anaphylaxis is so severe that a person's blood pressure drops and leads to shock. Shock happens because the blood vessels become larger and leaky, so oxygen is not able to reach vital organs. This can lead to heart attacks, strokes, and death. Anaphylaxis does not always progress to anaphylactic shock, but anaphylaxis should always be treated.

I want to reiterate that anaphylaxis does not require low blood pressure or throat closing! Identifying and treating anaphylaxis quickly before it progresses to those symptoms will significantly reduce the chances of severe complications developing.

The most common symptoms of anaphylaxis involve the skin, which is affected in 80 to 90 percent of cases. This is likely because the skin is home to a dense population of mast cells and other immune cells that are involved in a systemic allergic reaction. However, in cases of anaphylactic shock, it is estimated that 17 to 30 percent of cases did not involve the skin. This is probably due to low blood pressure causing a lack of blood supply to the skin.

When I am discussing anaphylaxis with my patients and their families, I provide them with a written plan that includes the signs and symptoms of anaphylaxis. While most plans that you find online will not say this, I often tell people that if you think you may have anaphylaxis, then it probably is anaphylaxis, and treatment should be started immediately. Calling a healthcare provider to verify whether someone is experiencing anaphylaxis could potentially waste precious time.

How Is Anaphylaxis Treated?

If you have experienced anaphylaxis in the past and know what the trigger is, avoiding the trigger is key. However, accidents can happen. I cannot stress this enough. If you suspect anaphylaxis, then epinephrine should always be used first. It is an injectable medication that usually comes as an auto-injector, and it works within a few minutes after injection. Epinephrine works by constricting blood vessels to help relieve upper airway swelling, low blood pressure, and shock. It can also open the lungs and improve the heart rate to move blood throughout the body.

The first needle-free device was approved in the United States in 2024 (it is also now available in the UK, Canada and the EU). It is called Neffy, which is a nasal spray containing epinephrine that is approved in the US for people ages four years and older weighing at least 15 kg. This device looks like Narcan (naloxone), a nasal spray used as an antidote for an opioid overdose. Neffy is a major advancement because many people are afraid to use needles on themselves or their loved ones. I will never forget prescribing Neffy for the first time. My patient was an adult who had recently become allergic to several foods and had multiple episodes of anaphylaxis shortly before I met her. She developed extreme anxiety toward eating and going out in public places. When I told her that the FDA approved Neffy, a wave of relief came over my patient's face. She was extremely scared of needles and it made her second-guess whether she needed to use epinephrine on multiple occasions.

Antihistamines such as diphenhydramine or cetirizine (Zyrtec, Piriteze) should not be used instead of epinephrine to treat anaphylaxis. Instead, antihistamines are used to treat milder symptoms such as itching, hives, and an upset stomach. Also, antihistamines cannot prevent anaphylaxis. This is because histamine is not the only substance that drives an anaphylactic reaction. Antihistamines are not able to quickly and effectively treat shock either. The faster epinephrine is used, the less likely that severe complications happen.

People living with asthma may be instructed by their doctor to take their rescue inhaler when anaphylaxis occurs to help with their breathing. One of the symptoms of anaphylaxis can be wheezing and this can be confused with an asthma attack. But if you suspect anaphylaxis, epinephrine should still be used first.

For years, healthcare professionals and patients in the United States have been taught that diphenhydramine (which is in the North American version of Benadryl) is the first choice for mild symptoms associated with anaphylaxis. People often choose Benadryl because of the myth that it works faster and is more effective than newer, second-generation antihistamines such as cetirizine (Zyrtec, Piriteze) and fexofenadine (Allegra, Telfast). Sometimes, people believe that diphenhydramine-containing US Benadryl is more effective because it makes them sleepy, but this does not mean it is treating or preventing anaphylaxis. There are multiple studies showing that second-generation antihistamines work as quickly as Benadryl, are just as effective, and last longer. Unless someone requires an intravenous antihistamine, where Benadryl is usually the only medication available, allergists are generally preferring a second-generation antihistamine over Benadryl for relief of hives and itching associated with anaphylaxis.

Education on anaphylaxis is crucial to help prevent this potentially life-threatening situation. Make sure your doctor has provided a written emergency action plan to help you recognize the signs of anaphylaxis and how to treat it. Please regularly review this document throughout the year and follow up with your doctor regularly to have the plan updated. Every auto-injector prescription comes with two devices and a training device that you can use for practice. If a training device is not in the box, you should call the manufacturer and request one. You should always carry two epinephrine devices in case you need an additional dose.

Call for help! Whenever you suspect anaphylaxis, emergency medical services should be called, even if someone is able to treat with an EpiPen or with a medication like Neffy. Not because epinephrine was used, but because anaphylaxis can be potentially life-threatening even after initial treatment, and monitoring may be necessary to watch out for biphasic anaphylaxis. While waiting for help, the person being treated should lie on their back with their legs elevated to help blood return to the heart. However, if they are not breathing well, then they need to remain upright and lean forward. Pregnant people and those who are vomiting should be placed on either side with their legs elevated. Propping an object like a pillow under their legs may help.

Keep in mind that newer clinical guidelines offer the possibility of managing anaphylaxis at home without going to the emergency room. However, this is not possible unless you talk with your doctors first and are well educated on the signs, symptoms, and treatment for anaphylaxis. I personally do not feel comfortable with any child experiencing anaphylaxis to be managed at home, but I am not here making this decision for you.

After emergency medical management concludes, it is important to follow up with your doctor to determine the trigger and to refill the epinephrine prescription. It may take multiple doctor visits to uncover the potential cause of anaphylaxis. You may want to wear a medical bracelet to instruct others in case of an emergency in the future.

In cases of idiopathic anaphylaxis, additional treatments are highly individualized. Whether someone is prescribed additional daily medications depends on the frequency and severity of the anaphylactic episodes. Additional medications that some doctors may prescribe include oral prednisone as an immune suppressant and antihistamine medications such as cetirizine and famotidine. Each anaphylactic episode should be discussed with a doctor to see if further information can uncover the potential trigger.

If you have ever experienced anaphylaxis, you know it can potentially cause a tremendous amount of stress and anxiety. I want you to ask yourself these questions:

Have you ever:

- Experienced intrusive memories of the traumatic event?

- Experienced nightmares about the traumatic event?

- Avoided places, people, or activities that remind you of the traumatic event?

- Experienced negative thoughts about yourself or other people?

- Felt detached from other people?

- Felt emotionally numb?

- Had trouble concentrating?

- Felt you were always on guard against danger?

- Felt easily scared or startled?

- Had trouble sleeping?

Many people who experience anaphylaxis may have symptoms of post-traumatic stress disorder. If you have experienced any of the symptoms listed above for at least four weeks or are having a hard time managing life, please talk with a doctor or mental health professional as soon as possible. You are not alone. Do not be afraid to ask for help. If you have suicidal thoughts, get help immediately. Call a suicide hotline.

Why Have EpiPens Been So Expensive?

Unfortunately, many people have not filled their epinephrine auto-injector prescriptions because they are too expensive. Most people are familiar with the EpiPen, which was approved by the FDA in 1987. Its market share rose to over 90 percent by the mid-2000s. In 2007, Mylan Pharmaceuticals received the rights to produce and sell EpiPens from the previous manufacturer, Merck. Mylan made several changes to the device to get new patents and help prevent generic versions of EpiPen being produced. During the next ten years, Mylan increased the price of the EpiPen from $94 to $609. Even with insurance, the out-of-pocket cost more than doubled from 2007 to 2014. In 2015, one of its main competitors, Auvi-Q, was temporarily recalled over dosage problems that led to serious safety concerns. This recall further strengthened Mylan's monopoly on the epinephrine device market. By 2016, a fraud investigation was initiated in response to public concerns about the high cost of the EpiPen. During that year, Mylan introduced a generic that was priced at $300 for a two-pack. In 2017, the fraud investigation concluded with a $465 million settlement of claims of improper Medicaid billing with no determination of liability.

Over the next several years, competitors entered the market and

Auvi-Q returned. However, the costs remained high for some people. A 2022 analysis from Chua and Conti revealed that from 2015 to 2019, average annual spending on epinephrine auto-injectors dropped from $115 to $75. However, about 8 percent of people were paying over $200 per year. Of those people, 63 percent were children. Those families were paying an average of $657 annually for their medication. This study found that the price was high not only for EpiPen but also for its competitors. Normally, generic medications are supposed to drive the cost down for a medication. However, EpiPen is a drug and device combination, so it is much more difficult for a generic alternative to get FDA-approved as an authorized generic alternative. Therefore, competitors set their prices near Mylan's $300 unbranded EpiPen.

For many families, the price gets out of control. Each prescription comes with two doses and a training device. It is recommended to always carry two devices in case a second dose is needed if symptoms do not improve within ten to fifteen minutes of the first dose. With children, they need a two-pack at school and at home. These devices also expire typically eighteen months from the date of manufacture. Some batches have been approved by the FDA for twenty to twenty-four months after expiration when there have been shortages. There is some evidence suggesting that the expiration date could be extended. A 2019 study published in *The Journal of Allergy and Clinical Immunology* reported that in a small batch of epinephrine auto-injectors, most devices retained 100 percent of their epinephrine content up to six months past the expiration date and over 90 percent of epinephrine content up to thirty months after expiration. Epinephrine is clearly expired if it shows signs of decay, which may include yellow discoloration, cloudiness, or the presence of particles. It is ideal to carry unexpired devices, but if there is a true emergency, using an expired device is probably better than not using epinephrine at all.

There has been pushback from lawmakers on the outrageous

price gouging of epinephrine auto-injectors. Multiple states, including Colorado, Delaware, Illinois, Minnesota, New Hampshire, New Jersey, New York, and Vermont, have signed laws that require insurers either to fully cover epinephrine auto-injectors or to cap the costs at anywhere between $25 and $100, depending on the state. In January 2024, the Epinephrine's Pharma Inflated Price Ends Now (EPIPEN) Act was introduced in Congress to try and cap epinephrine auto-injectors at $60 per twin-pack.

With needle-free alternatives becoming available, I am hopeful for the future that people will have better access to epinephrine. More people need it, and everyone should know how to use these devices. You never know when you may be able to save a life.

TAKE-HOME POINTS

- Anaphylaxis is a severe allergic reaction that can potentially be life-threatening.

- You do not need to feel your throat closing or a drop in blood pressure to experience anaphylaxis.

- The triggers for anaphylaxis are numerous and may not be identified in many cases.

- Epinephrine should be used first and quickly when treating anaphylaxis, but always follow up with medical treatment.

CHAPTER 13

Medication and Vaccine Allergies

Beth sat in the exam room of the urgent care, clutching a crinkled piece of paper with her medical records as she spoke to a doctor about her sinus infection. The doctor recommended prescribing a penicillin antibiotic called Augmentin (amoxicillin/clavulanic acid).

"My parents told me since I was a baby, I have been allergic to penicillin," she said. Her parents told her this story countless times. She had some kind of reaction as a baby after taking penicillin. It was severe enough in her parents' minds that she had never taken any penicillin antibiotics since then.

"Do you recall what happened specifically?" her doctor asked.

"I don't know. That was almost twenty years ago, and I was a baby, but that is all my parents told me," Beth replied.

What Is a Medication Allergy?

How many times have you been asked in a healthcare setting, "Are you allergic to any medications?" This is one of the most pervasive parts of healthcare, yet it is often riddled with misconceptions. Countless people are unnecessarily avoiding medications that they incorrectly believe they are allergic to.

An entire book can be written about allergic reactions to medications. My goal in this chapter is to help you gain a better understanding of what a medication allergy is, because misdiagnosing drug allergy is a growing public health problem. Some rare types of drug allergies will be covered to help raise awareness. Vaccines are considered a type of medication and will be discussed in this chapter as well.

Adverse drug reactions (ADRs) are any unintended and undesired effects of a medication. There are two main categories of ADRs, predictable and unpredictable. Predictable reactions usually depend on the amount of drug taken (i.e., dose) and the mechanisms of how the drug works, and they can theoretically happen in any individual. The vast majority of ADRs are predictable and include side effects, drug interactions, and overdose. Let's look at ibuprofen as an example. Ibuprofen is a nonsteroidal anti-inflammatory drug (NSAID) that is often used to treat fever and pain. A potential side effect is stomach pain, because ibuprofen is known to block chemicals called prostaglandins, which help protect the stomach lining from stomach acid. A drug interaction between ibuprofen and blood thinners such as warfarin (Coumadin) can increase the risk of bleeding. If too much ibuprofen is taken at once, overdose symptoms may include gastrointestinal bleeding, seizures, and coma.

Unpredictable reactions are less directly related to dose, are unrelated to the medication's underlying mechanism, and occur only in susceptible people. A medication allergy is an example of an unpredictable reaction that is due to an abnormal response to the drug by the immune system. There are many ways that the immune system can cause a drug reaction, and the reaction may happen immediately after taking the medication or it could be delayed. I will go over some examples throughout the rest of this chapter.

Penicillin Allergy—A Growing Public Health Crisis

Penicillin antibiotics are the most prescribed antibiotics in the United States. Examples include amoxicillin, ampicillin, nafcillin, and dicloxacillin. There are also combination penicillin antibiotics such as Augmentin, Unasyn (ampicillin/sulbactam), and Zosyn (piperacillin/tazobactam). Approximately 10 percent of Americans report having a penicillin allergy, but roughly 90 percent of these people do not have a true medication allergy. There are many reasons why this may be occurring.

As an example, people who have a "penicillin allergy" label may have experienced a rash or diarrhea when they took the antibiotic as a child. Their parents called their child's doctor, who erred on the side of caution and instructed them to avoid penicillin. The penicillin allergy label then sticks in the medical record for many years, unquestioned as to whether the symptoms were truly due to IgE-specific antibodies against penicillin. In previous chapters, we talked about anaphylaxis and symptoms of an IgE-mediated allergic reaction such as urticaria, angioedema, throat swelling, wheezing, difficulty breathing, vomiting, or low blood pressure. Many people experience diarrhea when taking an antibiotic because the balance of good versus bad bacteria in the gut is disrupted. That is a predictable side effect of penicillin and not an allergy.

The timing of the reaction helps indicate whether this is a true medication allergy, and the answers to these three questions may be helpful in determining if the symptoms are IgE-mediated:

1. Did the symptoms develop after the first dose?

2. Did the symptoms develop within one hour of taking a dose?

3. Did the symptoms resolve within one day of stopping the antibiotic?

If the answers to all three of these questions are yes, then there is a higher likelihood that the reaction was a true allergy. However, over time, the penicillin-specific IgE antibodies decrease. Roughly 80 percent of people with an IgE-mediated penicillin allergy lose their sensitivity to the antibiotic ten years after the reaction. Therefore, many people may carry the penicillin allergy label and not realize they have outgrown their allergy.

When a rash occurs while an infant or child is taking an antibiotic, it may not be a true medication allergy. The underlying illness may have been due to a viral infection, which can cause a rash, and was incorrectly attributed to the medication. Amoxicillin is also known to cause a rash in 5 to 10 percent of children, which is considered a side effect and not a true allergy. This type of rash usually starts three to ten days after the medication is started, and it consists of flat red patches that can sometimes be slightly raised. The rash often starts on the chest, abdomen, and back and then spreads to the face, arms, and legs. Symptoms typically last between one and six days. A rash is more concerning and likely to be a true allergy if it started within a few hours of taking the first dose and it is raised and very itchy. It may include swelling of the face or eyes, and it may be accompanied by other symptoms such as difficulty breathing, wheezing, or vomiting.

It is critical that people understand whether they are truly allergic to antibiotics, especially penicillin, because that label potentially leads to worse health outcomes. Penicillin antibiotics are the treatment of choice to combat many bacteria, including Group A streptococcus, Group B streptococcus, *Listeria monocytogenes*, *Neisseria gonorrhoeae* (gonorrhea), *Staphylococcus aureus*, and *Treponema pallidum* (syphilis). These bacteria commonly cause infections such as strep throat, skin and soft tissue infections, ear infections, pneumonia, sinusitis, acute rheumatic fever, and meningitis. A penicillin allergy label may lead to suboptimal treatment. For example, amoxicillin is recommended to help prevent surgical site infections for dental procedures, and alternative antibiotics are not as effective.

People who are allergic to penicillin are often given broad-spectrum antibiotics, which increases the risk of developing a *Clostridium difficile* (*C diff*) infection. That is a nasty gastrointestinal infection that leads to fever, stomach pain, and diarrhea. It also increases the risk of developing antibiotic-resistant germs, including methicillin-resistant *Staphylococcus aureus* (MRSA) and vancomycin-resistant *Enterococcus* (VRE).

Alternative antibiotics to penicillin are more costly and often cause more side effects. Vancomycin is an antibiotic often used as an alternative to penicillin, but it can cause damage to kidneys and severe allergic reactions. Overall, these issues may be the reason why a recent study estimated that the risk of death is increased by 14 percent in adults who have a penicillin allergy label.

Strategies for Addressing a Penicillin Allergy

While I have mainly been discussing penicillin to this point, many of these concepts apply to other ADRs (adverse drug reactions). If you ever have had a reaction to a medication such as penicillin, then it is crucial to record as much information as possible about the circumstances surrounding the reaction. The gold standard test for a medication allergy is to do a graded drug challenge, also known as test dosing. This is a cautious administration of the medication in a medically supervised setting. However, if the history of the reaction is recent and resembles an immediate, IgE-mediated allergic reaction, then testing may not be required.

Additional testing may be available to understand the risk of reacting to penicillin. Skin testing for penicillin and some important breakdown products of penicillin is one resource, but it may not be available or patients may not be able to stop their allergy medication to obtain it. There are clinical decision-making tools that help physicians determine the level of risk of reacting to penicillin. For example, there is the PEN-FAST tool, which has five criteria:

PEN: PENicillin allergy reported by patient
(if yes, proceed with assessment)
F: Five years or less since reaction (2 points)
A: Anaphylaxis or angioedema (2 points) **OR**
S: Severe cutaneous adverse reaction (2 points)
T: Treatment required for reaction (1 point)

If there are 0 points, then there is less than 1 percent chance of a true penicillin allergy. For 1 or 2 points, there is roughly a 5 percent chance of a true penicillin allergy. For 3 points, there is a moderate risk of a true penicillin allergy, roughly 20 percent, and 4 or 5 points is a high risk for a true penicillin allergy. This is a tool that can help identify the people who are at the lowest risk of having a true penicillin allergy and then performing a graded challenge to prove whether they are truly allergic.

For Beth, her PEN-FAST score was 0 because she had no recollection of what had happened to her, and she did not have any information from her parents surrounding the events that occurred when she was a baby. Therefore, she was given multiple small, incremental doses of amoxicillin in clinic and she had no reaction to the doses. She was relieved that she did not carry a penicillin allergy label anymore.

However, for some people, they may need to get penicillin even though they are truly allergic. When I was training in my allergy/immunology fellowship, I was consulted by the internal medicine team in the general wards of the hospital on a patient named Elmer. A few years earlier, he had developed facial swelling, hives all over his body, and wheezing within thirty minutes of taking his second dose of amoxicillin. He went to urgent care and was injected with epinephrine to stop his symptoms from progressing further. He had avoided penicillin antibiotics since then.

A couple of months before being hospitalized, Elmer developed blurry vision in his right eye. He went to his ophthalmologist, who did a series of examinations and tests, which revealed that he had ocular syphilis. When I met him, he was a generally upbeat man, but he appeared nervous. Elmer knew before I walked through the door that I was going to propose giving him the medication that had made him very sick a few years ago. It was clear that Elmer needed penicillin because it is the best medication to treat his ocular syphilis.

I discussed with him the process of penicillin desensitization, which is administering small, incremental amounts of the medication to temporarily induce tolerance to penicillin as long as the medication is taken without interruption. The desensitization wears off quickly if the medication is discontinued. In this case, I used penicillin G benzathine (Bicillin L-A), which is an intravenous form of penicillin used to treat ocular syphilis. Elmer was tense, but he was determined to get through the four-hour process. Every fifteen to twenty minutes, I was pushing incremental doses of the medication through his intravenous line. I sat with him the entire time while we watched fishing shows on the Discovery Channel. He was an avid fisherman, and I told him stories about fishing with my grandfather at Lake of the Woods near Winnipeg, Canada. He told me that he had some mild itching after a couple of doses, but he was able to tolerate the desensitization and was discharged home to complete treatment for the next couple of weeks.

What Are Serum Sickness and Serum Sickness–Like Reactions?

Mara was a bright, outgoing five-year-old who loved playing outside and exploring the world around her. She developed an ear infection after she recovered from a cold, which made her feel miserable for a few days. Her parents took her to their pediatrician, who confirmed that she had a double ear infection and prescribed amoxicillin for her. Within a few days, her ear pain was relieved, and she felt like herself again.

One week later, as she was finishing her antibiotic course, she woke up feeling miserable again. She had an itchy, red rash that was slightly raised throughout her arms, legs, chest, abdomen, and back. Mara was sweaty and felt hot to the touch. Her parents checked her temperature, which was 102.5°F.

"Daddy, my hands hurt!" she cried out. When her dad came close to her, he noticed that her hands and knees were swollen. Her parents called their pediatrician, who recommended that she get seen at their local emergency room.

Serum sickness is an uncommon allergic reaction to medications that is an example of the Gell and Coombs "type III" allergic reaction. The reaction occurs when an immune complex forms, which is when the medication and antibodies bind together to form a structure that can deposit into tissues such as joints. Immune complexes can activate other proteins, called complement proteins (not to be confused with a nice *compliment*), which perpetuate inflammation throughout the body. This leads to symptoms such as a fever, rash, and joint pain, which usually starts one to two weeks after the first exposure to the offending medication. Reactions to many medications may look like serum sickness but are believed to be caused by a different mechanism, which is referred to as serum sickness–like reaction (SSLR). Serum sickness is more common in adults, whereas SSLR is more common in children.

Mara was admitted to the hospital for observation and pain management. After the medication is stopped, treatment is focused on controlling pain with medications such as NSAIDs, and using systemic steroids for severe cases. Mara was given steroids intravenously because she had a high fever and severe knee swelling, making it difficult to walk. Within a few days, Mara felt like she was back to her normal self and was able to go home. From that point, she had to avoid penicillin and other similar antibiotics.

What Is Drug Reaction with Eosinophilia and Systemic Symptoms?

Micah had been a banker for the past thirty years and prided himself on staying active when he was not at work. Recently, he had developed gout and was prescribed a medication called allopurinol to help relieve the pain in his joints. At first, he was doing fine and was able to exercise pain-free again. However, after a few weeks of taking the medication, Micah developed a red rash on his abdomen and legs that was mildly itchy. His face became swollen as well. He called his doctor, who told him to come in as soon as possible. In the clinic, he had a fever and swollen lymph nodes in his neck. Micah's doctor ran some blood tests, which came back indicating a condition called drug reaction with eosinophilia and systemic symptoms (DRESS).

DRESS, as its name suggests, is usually an allergic reaction to a medication that leads to a fever, rash, elevated eosinophils, and organ damage. It is a rare drug reaction that occurs in about one in 100,000 people per year. While the underlying mechanism of DRESS is not fully understood, it is mainly considered a T cell–mediated allergic reaction. Its severity varies from a mild disease that can be treated at home with topical steroids when no significant organ damage occurs to a severe, potentially life-threatening situation in which multiple organs fail and high-dose steroids are needed in the hospital. Most people with DRESS recover completely, but it can take several weeks to months after the medication is stopped. DRESS survivors should be monitored for the development of autoimmune diseases because these complications can occur.

Micah had elevated eosinophils and signs of liver damage. His allopurinol was stopped, and he was given high doses of systemic steroids in the hospital. He was in the hospital for a couple of weeks, and he did not feel like himself again for three months. It was a long journey for him, and he contemplated retirement after the whole ordeal.

What Is Stevens-Johnson Syndrome and Toxic Epidermal Necrolysis?

Carmen was a bright and active woman who loved running. When she came down with a urinary tract infection, her doctor prescribed the antibiotic Bactrim (trimethoprim/sulfamethoxazole). Two days later, she woke up with a low-grade fever and a sore throat. She didn't make much of it at first, until that evening when her face felt like it was on fire. She could not fall asleep that night. Carmen looked in the mirror and noticed that her face was red. She tried putting moisturizing lotion on, but it made her face burn even more. Excruciating pain in her lips and cheeks set in, and she began to panic. The skin on her face was starting to peel off! Her husband drove her to the emergency room, and the doctors there became very concerned. They admitted her to the hospital for treatment for Stevens-Johnson Syndrome (SJS).

SJS and toxic epidermal necrolysis (TEN) are severe skin reactions where the skin becomes severely damaged and detaches, usually because of an allergic reaction to a medication, though some cases may not have a drug involved. This type of allergic reaction is mostly due to T cells abnormally attacking skin cells. SJS and TEN are classified based on the percentage of body surface area affected. When less than 10 percent of the skin is affected, it is classified as SJS, and when more than 30 percent is affected, it is called TEN. SJS/TEN overlap refers to when between 10 percent and 30 percent of the skin is affected. This is a rare disease that affects about one in 1 million people each year.

SJS/TEN not only causes severe skin damage, but it also can affect multiple organs. The skin helps maintain hydration and protects against infection, so people with SJS/TEN are at high risk of developing severe infections, dehydration, and electrolyte imbalances. Organ failure may also occur. Many people who develop this disease unfortunately pass away. Treatment requires multiple specialists to address the many problems that can arise from SJS/TEN.

Ultimately, treatment aims at healing the skin and preventing infections through wound care, managing fluid and temperature balance, and using medications that suppress the immune system. Fortunately, Carmen's SJS was caught early, and she received optimal care in the hospital for a few weeks before getting discharged home. Her vision became impaired, but her life was saved.

What Is a Vaccine Allergy?

Ellen spent countless hours in a busy emergency room, facing crises of all kinds. She was an emergency room nurse during the beginning of the COVID-19 pandemic, so she knew the dangers of SARS-CoV-2 well. When the first mRNA COVID-19 vaccines became available in December 2020, she was relieved that she would finally have some protection against this relentless virus. She was worried about bringing the virus home to her family, so she volunteered to be one of the first to get the vaccine at her ER, surrounded by familiar faces she trusted.

Within a few minutes of receiving her first dose, Ellen felt dizzy, her vision blurred, and her chest tightened. She was feeling short of breath and quickly called out for help. Her colleagues immediately evaluated her and found that the skin on her face and chest was red. They were concerned that she was experiencing a severe allergic reaction, so another nurse administered epinephrine, the lifesaving medication that she had used on other people numerous times before. Within a few minutes, Ellen's breathing returned to normal, and she felt much better.

Severe allergic reactions to vaccines are rare. As I mentioned before about other medications, there is a difference between an expected side effect of a vaccine and an allergic reaction. Most reactions to vaccines are temporary and relatively mild. The symptoms may last for a few hours to a few days, and commonly include pain or a rash at the injection site, mild fever, chills, fatigue, headache, joint pain, or muscle aches. Usually, these symptoms start within twenty-four hours after vaccination, but the symptoms may rarely appear a few days later. Some people may faint after getting a vaccine, which is also known as a vasovagal reaction. Panic attacks have also been reported after getting a vaccine, which may manifest as difficulty breathing and a fast heart rate.

An anaphylactic reaction to a vaccine usually occurs within thirty minutes after injection, but it can be delayed by a few hours. The rate of anaphylaxis to vaccines varies based on the vaccine, but its occurrence is rare. I have seen the rates range from 0.3 to 5 events per 1 million doses administered. While anaphylaxis can be potentially life-threatening, deaths attributable to an anaphylactic reaction to vaccines are very rare. A review of reports to the Vaccine Adverse Event Reporting System (VAERS) from 1990 to 2016 found that eight deaths may have possibly been due to an anaphylactic reaction to a vaccine in the United States. To put this in perspective, the National Weather Service reported that approximately twenty people die each year in the United States from lightning strikes.

There are several potential allergens in vaccines that could cause an anaphylactic reaction. Gelatin is found in the vaccines for measles, mumps, and rubella (MMR), varicella (chicken pox), and Japanese encephalitis (JE). Egg protein is in the yellow fever, MMR, and some influenza and rabies vaccines. However, the amount of egg is significant only in the yellow fever vaccine. People who are allergic to eggs can safely get the MMR, influenza, and rabies vaccines since the amount of egg protein is extremely small. Since the 2016–17 influenza season, the American Academy of Pediatrics has recommended that people with egg allergies receive any influenza vaccine. There are a small number of severely cow's-milk-allergic individuals who may react to the casein found in the vaccines that protect against diphtheria, tetanus, and pertussis (DTaP or Tdap vaccines). However, most people with a cow's milk allergy do not react to these vaccines. Some vaccine vial stoppers contain latex, which may pose a risk to latex-allergic individuals. The hepatitis B and human papillomavirus (HPV) vaccines contain yeast proteins, which could potentially cause a severe allergic reaction, but this is very rare. There may also be some trace amounts of antibiotics in vaccines, including neomycin, polymyxin B, and streptomycin.

If an immediate reaction to a vaccine causes concerns, then an allergist may perform skin testing with the components of the vaccine to help determine what may have caused the reaction and whether there is a risk of reacting to the vaccine in the future. In some cases, a vaccine may be given in small, incremental doses in a medically supervised setting to safely administer the vaccine.

Allergic Reactions to the COVID-19 Vaccines

When the mRNA COVID-19 vaccines were released in December 2020, there were reports of severe allergic reactions to the vaccine during the first few days that it was released to the public. In fact, there were six cases of anaphylaxis reported from the Pfizer-BioNTech mRNA COVID-19 vaccine after the first half million doses administered. There were also several reports of people experiencing "COVID arm," which was a large red, hot, itchy bump that appeared at the injection site. Initially, people were asked to wait fifteen to thirty minutes after vaccination to allow time for a reaction to occur because of concerns that many people were reacting.

Over time, we gained a better understanding of what was happening with these allergic reactions to the COVID-19 vaccine. When I saw Ellen in my clinic to evaluate her allergic reaction to it, allergists at academic institutions such as Harvard and Vanderbilt had recently published a suggested approach with skin testing done for components of the mRNA COVID-19 vaccine, which included polyethylene glycol (PEG) and polysorbates. I performed a skin test on Ellen using MiraLAX, methylprednisolone acetate, Refresh eye drops, and a hepatitis A vaccine. Her results were negative. It turned out that skin testing for components of the COVID-19 vaccine was not accurately predicting who would have an allergic reaction to the vaccine. In fact, many reports were coming out that for those who reacted to their first vaccine dose, the risk of reacting after the second dose was less than 1 percent. There may be two plausible explanations for this. First, many reactions may have been caused by a mechanism not due to an IgE antibody. An example of this is called complement activation-related pseudoallergy (CARPA). A pseudo-allergy is not a fake allergic reaction; it just means that it looks like an immediate allergic reaction, but the underlying mechanism is not due to IgE antibodies. Another hypothesis is a phenomenon called the immunization stress-related response (ISRR), which mimics an allergic reaction. ISRR is likely due to either anxiety or a stress response.

I spent a considerable amount of time discussing with Ellen whether she should get an additional dose of the COVID-19 vaccine. She was very nervous about getting another dose, but I reassured her that the likelihood of reacting was very low. Ellen thought about it for a while, and she realized that she needed to have additional protection against COVID-19. She needed to protect not only herself but her patients and family. As a precaution, I prescribed a prevaccination regimen of antihistamines, and she took the second COVID-19 vaccine in the emergency room among her peers. Ellen called me the next day and told me that she did not have any significant symptoms after the injection. We were all relieved.

As for "COVID arm," I saw at least one case almost every day for several months during the first half of 2021. Whenever a substance is injected, there is a risk that the immune system will respond to either the needle or the substance entering the body. This usually leads to a rash within the first one to two days after the injection. However, with the COVID-19 vaccine, this reaction does not usually appear until seven to eight days after the injection. The rash usually resolves within several days. Treatment is geared toward relieving inflammation, itching, and pain with cold compresses, topical steroids, oral antihistamines, and over-the-counter pain relievers.

I have spent a lot of time educating people about their health on social media. There is a lot of misinformation about vaccines on the internet that can sound confusing or even scary. However, do not let that be a substitute for information that comes from your doctor, who knows you well. If you have any questions or concerns, your doctor is one of the best resources to help in discussing the risks and benefits of vaccination.

TAKE-HOME POINTS

- Most reactions to medications and vaccines are expected side effects and do not mean that you are allergic to that substance.

- Document as much information as possible when a reaction to a medication occurs so that you can present the information to your doctor.

- Allergic reactions to vaccines are very rare!

CHAPTER 14

Mast Cell Disorders

This is the most difficult chapter for me to write. Mast cell disorders can be very confusing, and the research is constantly evolving. I wanted to make sure the information I present in this chapter is as accessible to as many people as possible. Many people are struggling with finding answers to their chronic ailments and have heard about mast cell activation syndrome (MCAS) on the internet. I hope this chapter will help provide more clarity. I had the opportunity to interview one of my followers from social media who told me a very powerful story about her life with MCAS. Keep in mind that her story—as well as the stories of others living with this condition—is unique. Please try not to compare yourself to her story if you are struggling with finding answers for whatever ails you.

Jane dealt with inexplicable health issues throughout her entire life. As a baby, she did not tolerate formulas well and vomited multiple times a day. She was colicky and constantly sick as a child, frequently seeing the doctor for common colds and ear infections. But at first, nothing seemed to raise any alarms for her family.

As she got older, she had trouble tolerating food. It seemed that anything she ate would cause her to have various symptoms, including intense stomach pains, nausea, diarrhea, chest pain, itching,

severe fatigue, and lightheadedness. Her relationship with food became increasingly fraught. At times, Jane felt as if her body had declared war on the very act of eating. Foods that were safe one day
could spark terrible reactions the next. She heard doctors saying that she had "food sensitivities" and "gut imbalances" and
offering her elimination diets. The tests her doctors obtained came
back with one elevated autoimmune marker, called ANA, which
provided some hope for Jane, but nothing definitive followed initially.

Jane's teenage years became more difficult. Her safe-food options dwindled to only a handful of choices—plain chicken, rice,
and some vegetables. The smell of certain foods would leave her
nauseated for days. She was plagued with hives, heart palpitations, and fatigue. It seemed as though her body was sensitive to
everything—temperature and altitude changes, exercise, and even
the pressure of certain fabrics on her skin.

One moment stood out sharply in Jane's memory. She was seeing her pediatrician, who she trusted and had hoped would find answers for her. Jane's pediatrician looked at her kindly, yet dismissively,
and said, "Jane, let's be realistic. You're not going to find something
that explains all your problems." Those words hit her like a ton of
bricks. Was she doomed to a lifetime of unanswered questions?
Would she ever get better?

The breakthrough came in 2020 near the beginning of the
COVID-19 pandemic. Jane went on a walk one chilly morning, only
to notice a strange sensation—her chest felt tight and her legs were
covered in itchy hives. Heart pounding, she felt the world spinning
around her. After a few hours, her symptoms dissipated, and she
was more determined than ever to get answers.

This time, she went to a gastroenterologist, who made a breakthrough. When Jane told him about her recent episode with hives,
she could see on his face that a light bulb came on. He ordered a test
for which she had to collect her urine for twenty-four hours in a container that would be shipped off to a lab for special testing. Sure

enough, it came back positive, and she finally started to get some answers.

What Are Mast Cell Disorders?

Mast cell disorders are illnesses where there are too many mast cells, they are hyperreactive, or both. There is a wide spectrum of problems associated with mast cell disorders. They can range from being somewhat harmless yet impacting quality of life to being potentially life-threatening or life-shortening. Remember, these cells often cause symptoms of allergic diseases, but they also play a role in wound healing and protect against parasites. They are located throughout the body but are highly concentrated in areas that interact with the external environment such as the skin, lungs, and gastrointestinal tract. Make sure that you review chapter 2 to go over some of the basic immunology concepts regarding mast cells. The concepts in this chapter may seem controversial to some people, but I will provide you with as much evidence as possible to help you learn more and navigate the issues.

These conditions may be broadly categorized as primary, secondary, and idiopathic mast cell disorders. I want to first introduce the concepts of these broad categories and then dive deeper into the specifics of some of these disorders. Mast cell activation syndrome was initially proposed to be a distinct idiopathic disorder in 2010. By 2022, a group of experts had expanded the definition of MCAS to become more of an umbrella term that encompasses primary and secondary mast cell disorders. Primary mast cell disorders are conditions where there is a defect in the population of mast cells that causes too many mast cells to be present or to become hyperreactive. It can be identified through specialized testing. The three conditions in this primary category are systemic mastocytosis (SM), cutaneous mastocytosis (CM), and monoclonal mast cell activation syndrome (MMAS). Secondary mast cell disorders are when the mast cells are normal in number and function, but they are responding to the environment in a way that causes unwanted symptoms. This is really a fancy way of describing most of the allergic diseases that have already been covered, such as allergic rhinitis, medication allergies, and physical urticaria. Essentially, if you have allergies, you can think of your condition as a form of abnormal mast cell activation. The third category is idiopathic mast cell disorders, those for which we cannot identify the underlying cause of mast cell activation. Examples include chronic spontaneous urticaria (chapter 10), idiopathic anaphylaxis (see chapter 12), and idiopathic mast cell activation syndrome. There are also conditions that increase the risk of developing mast cell disorders, such as hereditary alpha-tryptasemia (HaT).

Jane's gastroenterologist initially thought she may have had mastocytosis, but he was not an expert in mast cell disorders. At first, Jane tried finding an allergist or rheumatologist who understood these diseases, but she was turned away by multiple doctors because they either dismissed her symptoms or they did not feel comfortable trying to manage the complexities of her issues. After several months of searching, Jane found a specialist who was willing to see her, but she had to fly across the country for an appointment. Her parents, unwavering in their support, encouraged her to make the trip. "It's your decision," they told Jane. "Whatever you choose, we'll back you."

What Is Mast Cell Activation Syndrome?

MCAS is a condition in which someone experiences repeated episodes of symptoms of anaphylaxis or close to anaphylaxis. The underlying cause may or may not be known. When I talk to patients about MCAS, I often tell them that there may be too many mast cells present, or their mast cells may be twitchier than usual. However, we are not always sure why this is happening.

There are numerous potential triggers for MCAS symptoms, and they may change over time. They include sudden temperature changes, heat, cold, pain, emotional stress, pollution, exercise, food, alcohol, medications (e.g., NSAIDs, opiates), odors, perfume, infections, venom, sunlight, and mechanical friction. Many of these triggers can be unique to the individual, and allergy testing does not necessarily uncover them.

Mast cells release many chemical messengers, such as histamine, leukotrienes, prostaglandins, tryptase, interleukins, heparin, thromboxane, platelet-activating factor, and tumor necrosis factor. They do not always release the same chemicals when they are activated. Which chemicals are released depends on the type of stimulus and the signaling pathways that are activated. Since mast cells are found throughout the body, these mast cell mediators may cause several symptoms. Examples include abdominal pain, cramps, diarrhea, nausea, vomiting, bloating, skin flushing, urticaria, angioedema, itching, throat tightening, sinus pain, heart palpitations, difficulty breathing, wheezing, headache, brain fog, chronic pain, and fatigue. However, not all the symptoms I mentioned are a part of the diagnostic criteria for MCAS. Here are the consensus criteria that were developed in 2022, and all three criteria need to be met to be considered for an MCAS diagnosis:

1. Recurrent severe systemic symptoms in at least two organ systems consistent with mast cell-related symptoms. Symptoms may include:
   a. Skin: flushing, itching, urticaria, angioedema
   b. Respiratory: throat swelling, shortness of breath, wheezing
   c. Gastrointestinal: nausea, vomiting, diarrhea, abdominal pain
   d. Cardiovascular: rapid heart rate, low blood pressure, passing out

2. Significant transient increases in serum tryptase levels (preferably) or other mast cell-derived mediators over baseline during a period of increased symptoms.

3. A significant improvement in symptoms using medications that counteract mast cell mediator effects.

The reason why neurological and musculoskeletal symptoms are not included in the diagnostic criteria for MCAS is because while they are commonly reported symptoms, they are not exclusive to MCAS. It is important to make an accurate diagnosis because many diseases have features similar to MCAS. The differential diagnosis, meaning the list of possible conditions that could be causing symptoms, is extremely large. Here is a general overview of some of the possibilities, but this list is not comprehensive:

- **Cardiovascular:** heart attack, pulmonary embolism, endocarditis, deconditioning, orthostatic hypotension

- **Endocrine:** thyroid disease, adrenal insufficiency, carcinoid, pheochromocytoma, estrogen or testosterone deficiency

- **Gastrointestinal:** inflammatory bowel disease, irritable bowel syndrome, eosinophilic gastrointestinal diseases, gastroparesis

- **Rheumatologic:** vasculitis, systemic lupus erythematosus, erythema nodosum

- **Infectious disease:** viral, bacterial, parasitic infections

- **Neurologic:** epilepsy, dysautonomia, migraines, stroke, psychiatric conditions

- **Skin:** hereditary angioedema, rosacea, drug rash

While that list looks daunting, many of those conditions are rare. We do not know how often MCAS occurs, and I have seen estimates that vary significantly. I have seen rates reported as less than one in a thousand to as high as one in six people. It is very difficult to define how common MCAS is, given our current understanding of mast cells and the diagnostic testing that is available. I will discuss more about MCAS later in the chapter after we review some of the other mast cell disorders.

What Are Mastocytosis and Monoclonal Mast Cell Activation Syndrome?

Mastocytosis is a group of rare diseases where there is an abnormal accumulation of mast cells in the body. Cutaneous mastocytosis (CM) is when the accumulated mast cells are confined to the skin, while systemic mastocytosis (SM) is when other parts of the body are also involved. Roughly one in ten thousand people have mastocytosis. Most cases of SM occur in adults, while most cases of CM occur in children. CM often improves or resolves during puberty.

While we do not fully understand the underlying causes of mastocytosis, some genetic variants have been identified. There is a gene called *KIT* that is important for the development of mast cells, and the most common mutation of this gene that can be tested in commercial labs is the D816V mutation. This causes the development of more mast cells than usual. This mutation is not usually inherited or passed down from generation to generation.

There are multiple types of CM based on the appearance of the rash. The rash is usually reddish-brown patches that may be slightly raised. There may be one lesion or multiple lesions throughout the body. If the rash is lightly rubbed or scratched, it may produce a hive over the area, which is known as Darier's sign. A skin biopsy may be needed to confirm the diagnosis.

The World Health Organization has diagnostic criteria for SM. The diagnosis can be made if one major criterion and at least one minor criterion are present or if there are three or more criteria present:

1. **Major Criterion:** Biopsy of bone marrow or other organs that reveals ≥15 mast cells located near each other

2. **Minor Criteria:**
   - Biopsy of bone marrow or other organs where more than 25 percent of the mast cells have an abnormal shape
   - A mutation at codon 816 of the *KIT* gene in the bone marrow, blood, or other organs
   - Mast cells that express CD25, which is a protein found on the surface of some cells that are associated with SM
   - A blood total tryptase level that is persistently more than 20 ng/mL

I wanted you to see what these criteria look like to show you how much we understand mastocytosis. There is a lot of testing that needs to be done to determine whether someone has SM, and it can become time consuming and expensive and may require multiple specialists to obtain the tests. SM has multiple subtypes that are beyond the scope of this book, but some examples include indolent systemic mastocytosis, aggressive systemic mastocytosis, and mast cell leukemia.

To make things more confusing, MMAS is basically SM but does not fully meet the criteria for SM. There may be only one or two minor criteria for SM present. MMAS was first described in 2007, but it can be especially difficult to diagnose because of the complexity of obtaining the right bone marrow specimen to identify changes in the mast cells.

Jane spent almost two weeks while she was in college seeing the mast cell specialist. Because her evaluation was occurring during the beginning of the COVID-19 pandemic, she had to quarantine for several days after the flight before she could get tested over multiple days. She poured herself into preparation for this appointment, reading this doctor's book on mast cell disorders cover to cover. She underlined passages and filled the margins with notes. Jane felt that every page explained a piece of her life.

What Is Hereditary Alpha Tryptasemia?

HaT is a genetic trait that is autosomal dominant, meaning that there is a 50 percent chance for a child to inherit the trait if one parent has HaT. Roughly 5 percent of the population in the United States and Europe has HaT, which means there is an increased number of copies of the *TPSAB1* gene, leading to an increase in the production of a protein called alpha-tryptase. Tryptases are serine proteases, which are enzymes that cut into other proteins. Alpha-tryptase has numerous functions, but they mostly promote inflammation.

Surprisingly, most individuals with HaT either have minimal symptoms or have no symptoms at all. HaT is often seen in association with other conditions such as SM, idiopathic anaphylaxis, and stinging insect venom hypersensitivity. While there have been some reports of associations between mast cell disorders and irritable bowel syndrome (IBS), hypermobility syndromes such as hypermobile Ehlers-Danlos syndrome (EDS), and postural orthostatic tachycardia syndrome (POTS), there has not been definitive evidence that these conditions are linked to HaT.

Testing for HaT should be considered when tryptase levels are elevated. A genetic test can be obtained that will measure the number of copies of the *TPSAB1* gene. Treatment is usually not needed for HaT unless there is another underlying condition occurring. As an example, if someone has venom hypersensitivity, then venom immunotherapy may need to be lifelong (see chapter 16).

Challenges with Diagnosing Mast Cell Disorders

Measuring tryptase in the blood is the most specific test for mast cell activation. Ideally, a tryptase level should be obtained when someone is feeling well so that a baseline can be established to compare to additional levels. Mast cell activation is considered likely when subsequent tryptase levels increase greater than 1.2 x baseline value + 2 ng/mL. Ideally, this blood draw should be done within four hours of symptoms developing, which can be challenging. Another blood draw should occur after the symptoms have normalized, to help differentiate mast cell activation and mastocytosis. Allergy medications do not affect the tryptase level. This is the one test that is widely available at most commercial labs. However, if someone is sick enough to be in the emergency room, a tryptase may not be drawn by the emergency room physicians because they do not routinely interpret these tests, which take several hours to get results. I typically ask my patients to hold on to a prescription that requests this test to be performed and sent to me if they end up in urgent care or an emergency room.

There are other chemicals released from mast cells that can be measured, such as histamine, N-methylhistamine, prostaglandin D2, and leukotriene E4. These chemicals can be measured from a urine sample that is collected over twenty-four hours, but these tests present several challenges. Several of the chemicals are released not only from mast cells but also from other cells in the body. Tryptase is a more specific test for evaluating mast cell disorders. There are several factors that may influence the test, including how the sample is stored as well as bacteria in the urinary tract. These urinary tests do not have well-validated thresholds to determine a diagnosis. A test is generally considered positive if the results are significantly higher than baseline when the patient is feeling ill. Collecting and sending off urine can be complicated. You must make sure that the collection is in a container already chilled and that it remains cold for the entire collection period. The test that was positive for Jane on multiple occasions was the twenty-four-hour urinary N-methylhistamine test. This is a breakdown product of histamine that is mostly released from mast cells.

Many of the tests besides the one for tryptase are not available in many commercial labs, which makes it difficult not only for people to get access to these tests but also for physicians to know how to order and interpret them. Unfortunately, it can get expensive, especially since the tests may need to be done multiple times. Bone marrow biopsies may also be needed if SM is suspected.

Mast Cell Disorder Treatments and Management Strategies

Jane's experience working with her mast cell specialist over a few days became a turning point, after years when she had felt dismissed and not taken seriously. He had meticulously listened to all her concerns and pored over the tests. Everything seemed to line up with idiopathic MCAS as her diagnosis. She did not want to have a bone marrow biopsy because she was afraid of the risks associated with the procedure, so she was not sure if mastocytosis was a possibility. However, for the first time in her life she felt seen. The question remaining in her mind was, How was she going to feel better?

The first step in managing mast cell disorders is making sure that similar conditions that mimic mast cell disorders are excluded. As mentioned previously, there are many diseases that appear like mast cell disorders. It is challenging to differentiate all these diseases, and some people may argue that the diagnostic criteria for MCAS are too strict. In fact, one study of 100 people with suspected idiopathic MCAS found that only two people fulfilled all three of the diagnostic criteria for MCAS. There is a need for better access and easier tests for mast cell disorders.

People must figure out what are triggers for mast cell activation. Many of these triggers were previously mentioned, but I want to stress that it can take a long time to figure out what the potential triggers are for an individual. Sometimes, what was considered safe may become problematic later, and some triggers may fade away. Special attention needs to be paid whenever someone has a surgical or dental procedure, imaging studies that use contrast media, or vaccines. Additional medications may be given during these periods to help prevent mast cell activation. Women with MCAS may experience fluctuations in their symptoms that align with their menstrual cycle because the changes in estrogen and progesterone may have a direct influence on their mast cells.

Stress is a potent activator of mast cells. When someone says "it is all in your head," that is very dismissive. However, there is a physiologic basis for physical or emotional stress leading to mast cell activation. When stress occurs, a hormone called corticotropin-releasing hormone (CRH) is released from the hypothalamus in your brain, which eventually leads to release of the stress hormone cortisol from your adrenal glands. CRH and other substances can directly activate mast cells. Therefore, I strongly encourage anyone who has a mast cell disorder, or is suspected of having one, to seek mental health services to learn coping strategies for stressful situations. Symptoms of mast cell activation can appear quickly, unpredictably, and ferociously, like a tidal wave. People must learn how to mentally ride those tidal waves of symptoms so that they can recover quickly.

Even if a mast cell disorder has not been definitively diagnosed, there are various medications that can be used. Keep in mind that since the clinical definitions of mast cell disorders have evolved rapidly over the past several years, the effectiveness of these treatments for some of these mast cell disorders is not well defined and is being actively studied. To effectively study a treatment for a disease, the disease must be well defined so that the study population includes the appropriate people. Otherwise, it is difficult for your healthcare provider to know if a treatment can be applied to their patients. This means that treatments become highly individualized and experimental for many patients with mast cell disorders. In the United States, many of these treatments are not approved by the FDA, so insurance may not cover some of them.

The exception to what I have just mentioned is that the FDA has approved multiple medications for different types of SM, and which are available worldwide. There is a class of medications called tyrosine kinase inhibitors that help slow the growth of mast cells. Some of these medications are used to treat leukemia. Avapritinib (Ayva-kit) is a targeted treatment approved for adults that blocks the *KIT* D816V mutation. Midostaurin (Rydapt) blocks multiple targets in-cluding *KIT* D816V. While imatinib (Gleevec) is known to treat chronic myeloid leukemia by blocking Bcr-Abl tyrosine kinase, it also blocks other tyrosine kinase enzymes, including c-Kit, which controls mast cell growth. There are multiple potential side effects and risks associated with these medications, which should be dis-cussed with your doctor.

Anyone who has experienced suspected or confirmed anaphy-laxis should always carry epinephrine with them and learn how and when to use these devices (see chapter 12). Two devices should al-ways be with you in case you need a second dose. While Jane had never experienced confirmed anaphylaxis, she always carries epi-nephrine with her as a precaution. Remember, anaphylaxis is not a requirement to be diagnosed with MCAS.

Several medications that can block the effects of chemicals re-leased by mast cells are not only therapeutic but also diagnostic. If someone feels significantly better while taking these medications, then it may be a sign that they have MCAS. Second-generation H_1 antihistamines such as cetirizine (Zyrtec, Piriteze), levocetirizine (Xyzal), fexofenadine (Allegra, Telfast), and loratadine (Claritin) can be used to help treat itching and urticaria. The gastrointestinal symptoms may be alleviated by medications such as famotidine (Pepcid, Pepzan) or cimetidine (Tagamet). While they act as antac-ids, their underlying mechanism is H_2 antihistamine. Cromolyn so-dium is a medication that helps stabilize the mast cell membrane to prevent release of its contents. It comes in multiple preparations. When it is taken as an oral solution (Gastrocrom), it may help relieve gastrointestinal symptoms associated with mast cell activation. Gas-trocrom is taken four times a day, typically about fifteen minutes before a meal. This medication must be taken several times a day because it lasts only for a short time in the body. I must warn you, as much as this medication may help prevent symptoms associated with eating food, starting Gastrocrom can be challenging. If you start at a higher dose, it can cause significant diarrhea, so the amount taken needs to be slowly increased for the body to get used to it.

If symptoms are not improving despite taking antihistamines and cromolyn sodium, then antileukotriene medications may be considered. The most prescribed medication in this class is montelukast (Singulair), which may help alleviate breathing problems, itching, urticaria, or abdominal pain. The concerns regarding neurological side effects were addressed in chapter 11. Zafirlukast (Accolate) and zileuton (Zyflo) are other antileukotriene medications that are not widely used anymore because of the potential risk of severe liver toxicity. If these medications are used, then regular blood work must be obtained to monitor for liver damage.

Other treatment options have been investigated, but only case reports have been published, so it is difficult to determine whether they will be successful for people. For example, a middle-aged female developed MCAS, POTS, and restless legs syndrome (RLS). She also had evidence of small intestinal bacterial overgrowth (SIBO), which meant there was an excessive number of bacteria in her digestive tract. This can lead to abdominal pain, bloating, constipation, and foul gas. She was given a combination of low-dose naltrexone (LDN), intravenous immunoglobulin (IVIg), and antibiotics. Naltrexone is normally indicated for alcohol use disorder or opioid use disorder and blocks the effects of opioids. LDN is a significantly lower dose compared to the usual indications, and it may have positive effects for people with MCAS by decreasing cytokines from T cells that directly cause mast cell activation. This is one of the many potential mechanisms of how LDN is used to treat various disorders such as fibromyalgia, complex regional pain syndrome, and rheumatoid arthritis. IVIg may help in multiple ways—blocking histamine, increasing T regulatory cell activity, and/or blocking IgG receptors found on mast cells. Omalizumab has been used to treat MCAS and will be covered in more detail in chapter 17.

Over the course of a few years, Jane's condition has been relatively stable, but she has felt uncertain about her health. She feels good on most days if she adheres to her carefully crafted routine, avoids triggers, and maintains her medication regimen. Jane has been aware that MCAS can be unpredictable, and flare-ups are always a possibility. Despite these challenges, she has remained positive and grown strong through her self-advocacy and working with several doctors to navigate her chronic illness.

TAKE-HOME POINTS

- Mast cell disorders are illnesses where there are too many mast cells, they are hyperreactive, or both.

- Diagnosing mast cell disorders can be very challenging, likely requiring multiple rounds of testing and specialists to understand what is going on.

- Treatment of mast cell disorders is highly individualized and likely requires mental health services.

Part Three

Treatment Options

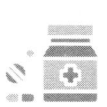 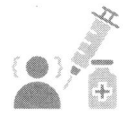 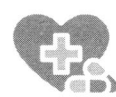

CHAPTER 15

Over-the-Counter and Prescription Medications

I f you have read the entire book up until this point, then you should be proud of yourself! We have covered so many topics, and the breadth of allergic diseases discussed is more than what most students learn during medical school. This last section of the book will go into more detail about specific treatments for allergic diseases and where the field is going from here. This chapter will focus on specific over-the-counter (OTC) medications, and I will discuss their potential risks and benefits.

I want to remind you that the treatments reviewed in this book are not specific medical advice to you. This book is meant to help provide general education about complicated issues and help guide you when you have conversations with your general practitioner about your health. Some prescription medications have been covered previously, but some important concepts will be explained here. Chapter 17 covers a class of medications called biologics.

Oral Antihistamines and Why It Is Time to Move on from Diphenhydramine

Oral antihistamines are medications that are often used to treat symptoms of allergic rhinitis, conjunctivitis, insect bites, urticaria, angioedema, and itching. They are sometimes used to treat nausea, vomiting, motion sickness, and insomnia in the short term. These medications prevent histamine from binding to the H1 receptor and work within fifteen minutes to two hours. When people ask me which oral antihistamine is the best for them, I respond with "What do you like better, Coke or Pepsi?" It is difficult to know which oral antihistamine is best for you, and you may need to experiment with each medication for a couple of weeks at a time. There are potential risks as well as benefits, which we will discuss at length in this section, which is why many doctors are moving away from regularly recommending older antihistamines.

What is the first medication that comes to your mind when you think about treating an allergic reaction? For many people in the US and Canada, it is diphenhydramine, where it is known as Benadryl, because it is one of the oldest antihistamine medications. Diphenhydramine became available in 1946 and is known as a first-generation antihistamine. Other examples include doxylamine (Unisom, Restavit), chlorpheniramine (Coricidin, Chlor-Trimeton), hydroxyzine (Atarax), dimenhydrinate (Dramamine), and doxepin (Silenor). At that earlier time, medications did not have to go through rigorous testing to evaluate their safety and efficacy, yet many people have been taking Benadryl throughout their lifetime. It is a relatively inexpensive medication that is often the go-to to treat allergic rhinitis, itching, cough, and urticaria.

However, the list of potential side effects is significant. Diphenhydramine can cross the blood-brain barrier and block histamine from binding to H1 receptors. This can cause significant drowsiness, which is why it is often used as a sleep aid. However, while you may fall asleep faster after taking diphenhydramine, it does not necessarily improve the quality of your sleep. Because diphenhydramine can linger in your blood for many hours, you may feel sleepy during the following day. It may even feel like you are hungover the next day. Diphenhydramine can impair your concentration and increase your risk of getting into a motor vehicle accident. In fact, there was a study of forty drivers who had allergic rhinitis, and the researchers reported that the drivers' performances in a simulation vehicle were worse when they took Benadryl rather than a placebo or fexofenadine (Allegra, Telfast), or when their blood alcohol level was approximately 0.1 percent (the legal limit in most states is 0.08 percent). This is why the Federal Aviation Administration does not allow pilots to fly until sixty hours after taking Benadryl or Unisom.

There are other side effects associated with taking Benadryl. You can experience dry mouth, dizziness, or feeling unsteady on your feet. At higher doses, it may cause blurred vision, urinary retention, impotence, nausea, constipation, and delirium. Some people may experience a phenomenon called paradoxical excitation, where instead of experiencing drowsiness, they experience insomnia, irritability, and hyperactivity. We do not understand why this happens, but one hypothesis is that some people may metabolize diphenhydramine differently, producing chemicals that are more excitable. Older age increases the risk of developing these side effects. You can overdose from taking too much Benadryl, which can lead to psychosis, seizures, and coma. Benadryl can cause death as well because of its potential for altering the heart's electrical activity.

Benadryl can also lead to hallucinations. Since the early 2000s, there have been message boards, blogs, and social media posts talking about the "Hat Man," also known as the "Benadryl Man," which is a tall, dark silhouette of a man in a brimmed hat, like the figure of Freddy Krueger from A Nightmare on Elm Street. I am not sure how this started or why the image is a man in a hat. People sell T-shirts online with the phrase "I can't take Benadryl because I owe the hat man money and I don't want to see him." In recent years, there have been social media trends that encouraged people to take high doses of Benadryl to experience hallucinations while on camera. This has been referred to as the "Benadryl challenge." Unfortunately, people have died after being encouraged to participate in this challenge, which prompted the FDA to issue a statement in late September 2020 warning people not to participate.

One of the potentially concerning side effects of taking a first-generation antihistamine such as diphenhydramine is its potential risk of cognitive effects. Because of its sedative effects, it can impact a child's ability to learn in the classroom. Medications like diphenhydramine are not only antihistamines, they are also anticholinergic medications. That means the medication can block the effects of a neurotransmitter called acetylcholine. This chemical messenger is involved with various brain functions, including learning, memory, attention, and focus. Anticholinergic medications are used to treat many diseases, including urinary incontinence, depression, and Parkinson's disease. There have been several studies showing an association between long-term anticholinergic medication use and developing dementia. However, establishing that anticholinergic medications cause dementia is very difficult. Clinical trials to establish causation would be very unethical to do. Can you imagine providing informed consent for a study that asked you to take a pill every day for many years, not knowing what you were taking or that it could potentially cause you to have dementia? I doubt many people would want to sign up for that study. Instead, we must infer based on observational studies that look at similar groups of people and whether they took anticholinergic medications chronically to see if they developed dementia later in life.

Most studies have not included Benadryl in their list of anticholinergic medications. There was one study from the University of Washington's School of Pharmacy that tracked roughly 3,500 people age sixty-five and older for an average of seven years and examined their medication records over the previous ten years. During the study period, 800 of the participants developed dementia. The study reported that taking an anticholinergic medication—which included first-generation antihistamines—for an equivalent of three or more years was associated with a 54 percent higher risk of developing dementia than taking the same dose for three months or less. Keep in mind that as you age, your body clears medications more slowly, so these older study participants were likely exposed to more medication. There may have also been interactions with other drugs they were taking, which can either increase or decrease the levels of anticholinergic medications in their bodies. It is unclear how much of an effect chronic Benadryl use has on younger people. While there is evidence that chronic Benadryl use may be associated with developing dementia, there is not enough evidence to say that it causes dementia. Fortunately, there are second-generation antihistamines that do not have anticholinergic effects, so if you are concerned about the potential cognitive risks, you have other options.

The second-generation antihistamines that are available are less likely to cross into the brain and do not have significant anticholinergic effects. Examples include Zyrtec, Piriteze (cetirizine), Allegra, Telfast (fexofenadine), Claritin (loratadine), and Xyzal (levocetirizine). There is a myth that Benadryl works more quickly than second-generation antihistamines, but multiple studies have reported that second-generation antihistamines such as Zyrtec, Piriteze and Claritin have a faster onset of action, increased potency, and longer duration of action to treat allergic rhinitis, urticaria, and food allergic reactions than first-generation antihistamines. In addition, for the treatment of chronic urticaria, you can safely increase the dose of second-generation antihistamines fourfold with your doctor's approval, which is not necessarily safe when using first-generation antihistamines. Keep in mind that any antihistamine medication has the potential long-term risk of weight gain. However, I am not aware of any study that helps determine which antihistamine medication carries a higher risk of weight gain. Also, stopping chronic use of antihistamine medication cold turkey carries a risk of developing severe itching, which is a rebound effect.

Slowly decreasing the amount of medication taken helps reduce the chances of this phenomenon occurring.

It is not a big deal if you take diphenhydramine occasionally. In fact, if there is an emergency where an antihistamine is needed to be given intravenously, then diphenhydramine is sometimes the only option available. However, I do not believe that everyone is fully aware of their options. There is enough evidence, when you weigh the risks and benefits of taking diphenhydramine compared to second-generation antihistamines, that for most people it is time to move on.

Intranasal Steroids and Antihistamines

Regardless of whether you have allergic rhinitis, non-allergic rhinitis, or allergic conjunctivitis, nasal sprays that contain either a steroid or an antihistamine are more effective than oral antihistamines, especially when it comes to treating nasal congestion and postnasal drip. This is one of the reasons why environmental allergy testing is important. If the testing is negative and someone has non-allergic rhinitis, then oral antihistamines may not be as effective as a nasal spray. There are several OTC nasal sprays that contain steroids (also known as intranasal corticosteroids—INCS), including Flonase, Flixonase (fluticasone propionate), Nasacort (triamcinolone acetonide), Nasonex (mometasone), Rhinocort (budesonide), and Flonase Sensimist, Avamys (fluticasone furoate). The only OTC nasal sprays available that contain an antihistamine (also known as an intranasal antihistamine—INAH) are Astepro, Rhinolast, Eze Allergy and Astelin (azelastine).

Is INCS or INAH better at treating nasal symptoms? Studies investigating this question reported conflicting results. While some studies showed that they are equally effective, other studies reported that INCS may be superior to INAH. One of the advantages of INAH is that it can work quickly, within fifteen to thirty minutes! INCS may take several days before you see the full benefits of these sprays, but this medication can significantly improve symptoms, especially when it is used chronically. However, INAH can have a bitter taste that lasts for several minutes. Other side effects may include headaches, nose bleeds, drowsiness, and throat and/or nasal irritation. To help minimize the chances of experiencing that bitter taste, I have shown people how to use a nasal spray properly: Make sure that you tilt your head down and point the spray slightly out toward your ear on the same side as the nostril, and do not snort the medication because not only will you be more likely to taste it, but you will also waste some of it. In other words, "If you taste it, you waste it!"

Now that azelastine is available OTC, it is easier to take both an INCS and INAH at the same time. Multiple studies have shown that combining an INCS with INAH is superior in reducing symptoms of allergic rhinitis and works faster than each individual component can accomplish. As Aristotle once said, "The whole is greater than the sum of its parts." While this method can be prescribed in the form of Dymista (fluticasone propionate and azelastine)—this is available OTC in the UK—or Rylatris (olopatadine hydrochloride and mometasone furoate), you can get the individual nasal sprays OTC for Dymista.

When a child or adult takes an INCS at recommended doses, there are not usually significant systemic side effects. However, there is a concern that children may have stunted growth if they take an INCS long-term. As an example, in a study randomized over 370 prepubescent children who took either Flonase Sensimist/Avamys daily or a placebo, there was an average difference in growth velocity of 0.28 cm per year when using an INCS versus a placebo. Therefore, if a child is taking an INCS for more than a couple of months, it may be best to have their growth monitored closely. The most common side effects of INCS are nasal irritation, dryness, and nose bleeds. In older people, chronic use of INCS may be associated with developing cataracts and glaucoma because of the small potential for a person's eyes to be exposed to the corticosteroids. However, this risk is most likely minimal.

Decongestants

Alex was busy managing a restaurant while training for an upcoming marathon, so there was no room for setbacks. When he developed a sinus infection, he could not seem to get his stuffy nose under control, so he found a quick fix at the pharmacy—Afrin. At first, it seemed to work like magic. With just two sprays, Alex could breathe again, free to power through the workday and long running sessions. However, as time passed, the nasal congestion stayed. "Must be allergies," he thought, so he continued to use Afrin every day to find similar relief.

Days turned into weeks, and Alex started to rely on Afrin to sleep. If he did not take the medication, his nasal congestion would return worse than before. Alex felt that something was wrong. He checked the instructions on the medication's box, and he was horrified to realize that he had forgotten to read the warnings, which stated that he should not take the medication for more than three days in a row. He went to an allergist for help.

It turned out that he had developed a condition called rhinitis medicamentosa. This is when a person uses a nasal decongestant spray such as oxymetazoline (Afrin, Dristan, Drixine, Demazin, Iliadin, Oxymist, and Sinex) or phenylephrine (Neo-Synephrine, Nazene, and some OTC cold and flu medications) regularly for many days, which causes rebound nasal congestion. A vicious cycle starts, where the medication causes nasal congestion and temporary relief but it eventually leads to a dependency on this medication. These nasal sprays should not be taken for more than five days in a row and should not be taken more frequently than recommended. There is some evidence that rhinitis medicamentosa is less likely to occur if an INCS is taken with a nasal decongestant. Treating rhinitis medicamentosa can be particularly challenging. The nasal decongestant must be stopped, and the nasal congestion is likely to get worse before symptoms improve. Switching to an INCS is usually required to treat the rebound nasal congestion. For Alex, a short course of a systemic steroid was prescribed to help because his congestion was very severe. However, it took him six months to fully recover. Sometimes, it can take as long as one year before a full recovery from rhinitis medicamentosa.

Even though I shared with you an example of how misusing a nasal decongestant spray can be harmful, these medications can be immensely helpful for quick relief of nasal congestion, whether it is from a cold or chronic rhinitis. These nasal sprays are becoming more important now because of the recent changes in what we know about oral decongestants.

You may have heard on the news that the FDA in 2024 recommended that the widely used oral decongestant phenylephrine should not be sold OTC anymore. Oral phenylephrine has been found in at least 250 products in the United States. Examples include Sudafed PE, DayQuil Cold & Flu, Mucinex Fast-Max Severe Congestion & Cough, and Theraflu ExpressMax Severe Cold & Flu. Any medicine that has "PE" in the name contains phenylephrine. In 2022, over 240 million items were sold that contained oral phenylephrine, which is $1.76 billion in revenue. However, for many years, pharmacists and doctors have known that oral phenylephrine is not effective at treating nasal congestion, so how did we get to that point?

In 1976, a review panel from the FDA concluded that oral phenylephrine, pseudoephedrine, and phenylpropanolamine were safe and effective nonprescription oral decongestants that could be used for allergic rhinitis, a common cold, and sinusitis. They all work by shrinking blood vessels in the nasal passages to reduce swelling. However, in 2000, phenylpropanolamine was removed from all products because strokes were reported after use. In 2005, the FDA created the Combat Methamphetamine Epidemic Act under Title VII of the USA Patriot Improvement and Reauthorization Act, which banned all OTC sales of pseudoephedrine (Sudafed) and required this medication to be sold behind the counter, meaning you had to show your identification card to a pharmacist before you could get Sudafed. This was because Sudafed could be used to create methamphetamines. Since then, the sales of oral phenylephrine have steadily increased to the point that in 2022, products containing oral phenylephrine were sold more than five times as often as the number of products containing Sudafed, because they were the only oral decongestant that was visibly available.

In 1971, an unpublished study by Hylan A. Bickerman of Columbia University reported that oral phenylephrine was not effective. Leslie Hendeles, Pharm D, from the University of Florida, published a review in 1993 agreeing that oral phenylephrine was not effective. Then, in 2005, Randy Hatton, Pharm D, contacted Dr. Hendeles and they started working together to determine whether oral phenylephrine was effective. They reviewed the existing medical literature on oral phenylephrine and found that it was no better than a placebo. This is because when phenylephrine is taken by mouth, it breaks down in the liver before the medication reaches the nasal passages. This does not happen to nearly the same extent if phenylephrine is formulated as a nasal spray. Oral phenylephrine was rarely sold prior to 2005, so it was not heavily scrutinized until these pharmacists petitioned the FDA twice to reevaluate the effectiveness of oral phenylephrine. In September 2023, an advisory committee for the FDA unanimously voted that the evidence supports the claim that oral phenylephrine is ineffective. The FDA is known to be an agency that focuses on the safety of medications, and since the safety of oral phenylephrine has not been questioned, it took several decades to acknowledge that oral phenylephrine is a useless OTC drug.

Fortunately, Sudafed is still available if you talk with your pharmacist. This decongestant may also be combined with antihistamines to provide superior relief. Examples include Claritin-D (loratadine-pseudoephedrine), Zyrtec-D (cetirizine-pseudoephedrine), and Allegra-D (fexofenadine-pseudoephedrine)—these are not available in the UK, though Sudafed and antihistamines are sold separately. The D stands for *decongestant*, which is always pseudoephedrine. Keep in mind that there are several side effects associated with using Sudafed, including high blood pressure, insomnia, irritability, and headache. It is best to avoid Sudafed if you have a history of high blood pressure or you are using a class of medications called monoamine oxidase inhibitors. Sudafed should be used with caution if you have hyperthyroidism, bladder neck obstruction, cardiovascular disease, cerebrovascular disease, or closed-angle glaucoma. While Sudafed is not associated with developing rhinitis medicamentosa, I am personally not a fan of taking Sudafed regularly, because it may cause nervousness, dizziness, persistent abdominal pain, vomiting, and raised blood pressure.

Cromolyn Sodium

Cromolyn sodium (NasalCrom, Nalcrom) helps stabilize mast cells to reduce the release of histamine and other chemical messengers that promote inflammation. NasalCrom is available OTC as a nasal spray that is taken as one to two sprays at least three or four times a day. NasalCrom is well tolerated. (In the UK, cromolyn sodium is only available in capsule form, Nalcrom, with a prescription.) However, it is less effective than second-generation antihistamines or INCS. If you know what you are allergic to, then you can try taking it prior to being exposed to the allergens. For example, if you have an allergy to tree pollen, you need to start taking cromolyn sodium one to two weeks prior to the start of tree pollen season.

Eye Drops

There are several options for eye drops to treat allergic conjunctivitis. However, be careful when you are buying eye drops. In 2023, the FDA published several warnings regarding certain generic eye drops that were contaminated with bacteria due to unsafe manufacturing practices. At least eighty people were affected, with over a dozen people experiencing significant vision loss, and at least four people died from sepsis due to contaminated eye drops. Although eye drops are expensive, I do not believe it is worth looking for cheaper alternatives. Stick with well-known brands.

Artificial tears can help soothe dry eyes and help clean the eyes when they are exposed to irritants and allergens. I find that they feel better on your eyes when you store them in the refrigerator. There are two main categories of artificial tears—eye drops with preservatives and preservative-free eye drops (bottle may say "PF"). Eye drops with preservatives help prevent growth of bacteria after the bottle has been opened, but they may irritate your eyes when you use them. PF eye drops have fewer additives and are easier to use if you apply artificial tears multiple times per day, and they often come in single-dose vials. Examples of artificial tears include Blink Tears, Refresh Tears, Systane Complete PF Preservative-Free Dry Eye Relief, and Optrex Moisturizing Eye Drops.

Several eye drops containing antihistamines with mast cell-stabilizing properties are sold OTC. Examples include Pataday, Opatanol, Alcon (olopatadine), Lastacaft (alcaftadine), and Zaditor, Zaditen (ketotifen fumarate). Keep in mind that these eye drops may cause a temporary stinging or burning sensation because the active ingredients may have a slightly acidic or alkalotic pH level. They may also contain preservatives such as benzalkonium chloride that can contribute to irritation. There are also eye drops that combine an antihistamine with a vasoconstrictor that helps treat eye redness. Examples include Naphcon-A, Visine, and Opcon-A (Optrex Allergy and Optrex Red Eyes in the UK). These eye drops contain pheniramine, which is the antihistamine, and naphazoline, which is the vasoconstrictor. However, naphazoline can cause the rebound redness that we talked about earlier with rhinitis medicamentosa. You should not use these eye drops for more than seventy-two hours.

Several eye drops are available by prescription only. An example of a prescribed allergy eye drop is azelastine hydrochloride, which acts as an antihistamine and mast cell stabilizer. There are also steroid eye drops such as loteprednol etabonate (Alrex, Loteflam, Lotemax). However, steroid eye drops should be monitored closely because there are several side effects that may occur, such as blurry vision, increased risk for eye infections, and increased eye pressure that can lead to glaucoma and vision loss.

Nasal Saline Rinses

Rinsing the nasal passages with saline water is frequently used to treat chronic rhinitis and sinusitis. It can help clear out irritants, allergens, and mucus to help moisturize the tissue as well as allow nasal sprays to work more efficiently. Nasal mucus acts like flypaper and traps as many particles as possible, so that needs to be removed first to help the nasal spray medication get to where it needs to be. There are several methods for delivering nasal saline, including a nasal spray, bottle, nebulizer, pump, or pot. The ideal amount of salt in the solution has not been definitively established. Rinsing the nasal passages can be difficult to do and there can be some side effects, including irritation, burning, and nausea. It takes several steps to complete, and the delivery device may need to be cleaned regularly. Always make sure you read the instructions of the product carefully before using.

Tap water should never be used unless it is boiled for at least a minute and then cooled before use, to avoid transmitting bacteria and parasites. Every so often, you may have heard of someone developing a "brain-eating amoeba" infection, which refers to the parasite *Naegleria fowleri*, which is almost universally fatal. To avoid this potential risk, boil the water you use or buy distilled or sterile water. Always read the instructions carefully for nasal rinsing products and understand how to clean their delivery devices regularly.

Important Points Regarding Prescription Medications

Allergy and asthma medications that are prescribed can be very expensive! For those who have to pay for them, I have several suggestions to help reduce the cost of obtaining these medications. At the beginning of January each year, the medications covered by your insurance plan may change. Call your health insurance company to obtain a list called a drug formulary, which explains what medications are covered by your insurance plan. Once you have this list, you can let your doctor know what is covered so that time is not wasted sending multiple prescriptions to the pharmacy. In my experience, this is especially important for people who need asthma inhalers.

Ask your doctor to prescribe generic medications whenever possible because they are usually cheaper. Direct-to-consumer pharmacies may be able to offer generic medications at lower prices. Pharmaceutical companies may offer copayment cards or manufacturer coupons that can drop the cost of the medication, which is usually covered by private insurance. Your doctor may have these coupon cards, or they can be found on the manufacturer's website. Price comparison tools aggregate discount coupons and compare prices among pharmacies to help people find the lowest prices in their areas. There may be payment assistance programs available as well.

Final Thoughts on Medications

The allergy aisle in supermarkets and pharmacies has grown over the years, and choosing what products are right for you can be confusing. I encourage you to talk with your local pharmacist to make sure you understand which OTC medications may be right for you. They can help clear some of the confusion about these medications, and they are a great resource for showing you how to take specific medications. You may need to spend several weeks trying different OTC medications before some combination appears to be effective. However, if you are struggling with managing your symptoms on your own, then I highly recommend seeking medical attention. You may need prescription medications or other therapies to help, which may require close monitoring and follow-up.

TAKE-HOME POINTS

- Diphenhydramine, for most people, is not necessarily the best treatment for allergic diseases, especially if it is taken chronically.

- Nasal sprays containing corticosteroids or antihistamines are superior to oral antihistamines in treating nasal symptoms.

- Do not take nasal decongestant sprays containing oxymetazoline or phenylephrine for more than five days in a row because they increase the risk of developing rhinitis medicamentosa.

CHAPTER 16

Immunotherapy

At six years old, Aaron was already cautious around food. His parents instilled in him that he needed to avoid both peanuts and tree nuts because they were dangerous for him to eat. When he was a baby, he developed hives all over his body and vomited after eating peanut butter. Aaron was rushed to the emergency room and given epinephrine. A similar episode happened to him when he was three years old after he ate ice cream that contained pistachio. A constant fear weighed heavily on his parents. They did not want to see Aaron go to the emergency room again. Aaron lived in a world where peanut butter sandwiches and cookies were off-limits, which left him feeling different from his friends. Aaron had to sit at a separate table from them for lunch at school. He did not feel safe at school, and his parents were highly motivated to help him stay safe from food allergens however they could.

Chelsea had always loved cats. As a kid, she loved visiting her friends who had cats so she could play with them. She loved petting their soft fur and the sounds of their gentle purr. There was one problem—Chelsea was allergic to cats. Whenever she was around them, it felt like she was paying the price with sneezing, runny nose, and coughing. On rare occasions, she would hear a faint wheeze in her chest after playing with a cat. Her parents would not allow cats in their house. Now, as a young adult, she was dealing with allergies throughout the year and was getting tired of having to take a lot of medications to keep her symptoms at bay. She met with me to see what could be done about her chronic symptoms.

While these stories seem vastly different, there is one common thread between these two people: Immunotherapy may be used to help treat the underlying problem. This treatment helps train the immune system to become less reactive to an allergen through controlled, regular exposures to that allergen. Immunotherapy can be given through multiple routes, including via injection or ingestion. This chapter will discuss how immunotherapy may be used to treat food allergies and environmental allergies.

Oral Immunotherapy to Treat Food Allergies

One day, Aaron's mother was scrolling through social media and started seeing posts about oral immunotherapy (OIT) to treat food allergies. She was intrigued by the prospect of treating her son's food allergies, so she looked online and read more about OIT, and she came across a website called www.fastoit.org that listed allergists who offered this treatment. Aaron's family found me this way and set up an appointment to learn more.

I met Aaron's family and discussed his health history, reviewed his previous laboratory testing from two years prior, and discussed the potential risks and benefits of OIT. This food allergy treatment has been studied and implemented in many countries. The only FDA-approved OIT treatment is called Palforzia (*Arachis hypogaea*), which is used to treat peanut allergy in children ages one to seventeen. Palforzia has been available since 2020, and is also approved in the UK and EU. Many allergists and I have provided OIT for other foods since there are no other FDA-approved products. Some of the foods I have offered OIT for include peanuts, cashews, walnuts, sesame, eggs, and chickpeas.

The goal of treating food allergies is to induce tolerance of the food, meaning there is a permanent state where someone can eat the food allergen without reacting and can have periods of not eating the food and be able to safely reintroduce that food into their diet. Unfortunately, at the time of writing this book, there is no treatment—including OIT—that can reliably accomplish this goal. Instead, the realistic goal of OIT is to increase the amount of food allergen that can be consumed before causing symptoms. This process is also known as desensitization. Think of OIT as providing a protective coat against anaphylaxis. This process may significantly reduce the chances of developing symptoms if there is accidental ingestion. Over time, some people may be able to achieve a state called sustained unresponsiveness. This is a lack of reaction to a food allergen after active OIT is stopped for a period—usually weeks to months. However, there usually needs to be some level of continued exposure to maintain this state.

The process of OIT typically involves first taking very low doses by mouth, such as 3 to 6 mg of food protein. In my clinic, we administer the initial doses in the clinic as part of a "rapid escalation phase." Ten incremental doses are given roughly every twenty minutes, so the initial office visit is four to five hours depending on how fast the doses are administered. Then, doses are provided and given at home roughly at the same time each day. Every one to two weeks, patients return for a dose escalation visit that lasts for roughly one hour. If the higher dose is tolerated, then they are sent home with more doses to continue the process. It takes roughly five to six months to reach the "maintenance dose," which is the dose that is taken every day indefinitely. This maintenance dose and the time it takes to get there vary depending on the allergist you work with. In my clinical practice, the maintenance dose for peanuts is three peanuts a day (~750 mg peanut protein). The maintenance dose for Palforzia is 300 mg of peanut protein. However, I have met people who have been on much higher maintenance doses for peanuts, including one person who was consuming twenty-one peanuts every day!

Aaron's parents were very interested in OIT after learning about its potential benefits. They felt that it might take the edge off their daily anxiety over protecting their son. They did not want to feel like they were doing nothing to treat his food allergies. Only avoiding food did not sit well with them. Aaron's parents knew that Aaron would have to adhere to some strict protocols to safely administer OIT. It is possible to develop allergic reactions to the OIT doses. Risk factors for developing allergic reactions include taking a dose on an empty stomach, because the dose may be absorbed more quickly, causing the immune system to respond more robustly. Missed doses can increase the risk of reacting to an OIT dose. Illnesses, especially if a fever is present, may increase the immune system's reactivity to a dose. Taking a hot shower or exercising elevates the body temperature, which may also produce an allergic reaction. Therefore, a rest period must happen around the dose each day. In my clinical practice, we recommend a rest period of one hour before taking an OIT dose and two hours afterward.

I spent a considerable amount of time counseling Aaron's parents about the potential risks of OIT as well. Many side effects can occur because the doses contain food allergens. People commonly complain of itching, tingling, and swelling in the mouth and throat, which is usually mild and self-limiting, but it can be quite uncomfortable for some people. Abdominal pain, nausea, vomiting, diarrhea, urticaria, angioedema, coughing, wheezing, shortness of breath, nasal congestion, and sneezing may also occur. Anaphylaxis due to OIT doses can happen during the buildup or maintenance phases and require using epinephrine. Multiple studies have reported that anaphylaxis occurs more often in people undergoing OIT than those avoiding food allergens. Rarely, eosinophilic esophagitis develops during the OIT process. This is a type of inflammation that can cause symptoms of gastroesophageal reflux, difficulty swallowing, and food getting stuck in the esophagus. If this happens, then OIT must be discontinued. If someone has uncontrolled asthma, they cannot safely pursue OIT.

I do not believe OIT is helpful for everyone who has food allergies. The risks and benefits must be weighed carefully, and the family must be completely committed to the process. Also, OIT may not be covered by insurance, so the procedure can be costly. Aaron's family was highly motivated and understood the potential risks. They knew that Aaron could react to the doses, but they felt that their anxiety would improve if they could give him some protection. Before starting OIT, I recommended that we determine which tree nuts Aaron was allergic to since he had not been tested in a couple of years. It turned out that he was allergic only to peanuts, cashews, and pistachios. Therefore, his OIT regimen would consist of doses of peanut and cashew since cashew and pistachio are cross-reactive. Aaron would get protection from pistachio by being treated for cashew.

The first day of OIT was filled with nervous excitement for Aaron and his family. His first doses were diluted into a solution and were tiny, almost invisible, but they set off a chain of events that would change everything. He did not have any reactions to the ten doses that were given during the five hours in my office. At home, however, their lives had to adjust. Every evening after dinner, Aaron was given a dose of peanut and cashew. He struggled initially to take his doses, and he was not always happy—Aaron was not allowed to play sports outside or take a hot bath after his dose. Over time, he got used to taking his doses and showing up to the clinic for higher doses each week. There were a few times when he complained of an itchy mouth or a stomachache, but these symptoms were mild and quickly addressed each time.

Days turned into weeks; weeks turned into months. Tears filled his mother's eyes when she saw Aaron eat his first whole peanut and cashew. She thought it was not possible, but the hard work felt worth it. A few weeks later, Aaron finished the up-dosing phase. The process took him five months, just in time for his seventh birthday. He felt a sense of accomplishment, and his parents were relieved that he did so well. Eventually, he was allowed to replace his peanut dose with a snack-size Reese's peanut butter cup. While he still had to always carry an epinephrine auto-injector and still could not freely eat nuts, his family felt safer and less stressed when they went to restaurants or social events. Aaron had a quiet feeling of normalcy around his friends, and his family felt that they had a bright future.

Now, I do not want Aaron's story to feel like I am completely sugarcoating OIT. I have taken care of many patients who have successfully completed OIT and were protected against accidental ingestion of their food allergens. However, I have also seen patients who were either unable to complete OIT or stopped not long after completing the initial up-dosing phase. In my experience, the patients who are less likely to be successful are those who are unable to adhere to the guidelines that help reduce the risk of developing reactions or the patient is overscheduled. For example, if a patient is an athlete and has multiple late practices in a week, then they would have to wait an hour after practice to take their dose and then stay up for two additional hours to make sure no reactions occurred. Multiple studies have reported that younger children tolerate OIT with fewer symptoms than older children and adults. Teenagers and young adults may struggle with taking doses every day, especially if the patient has not completely bought into the OIT process.

OIT Protocols and Other Food Allergy Therapies Under Investigation

There are efforts to improve the safety and effectiveness of OIT. Multiple clinical trials have investigated whether the biologic medications omalizumab (Xolair) or dupilumab (Dupixent) can improve OIT. The studies are either small or ongoing, so these therapies are under active investigation. More information on these medications will be discussed in chapter 17. The administration of probiotics with OIT may reduce the frequency of allergic reactions to the doses. I have found that some of my patients who take probiotics with OIT experience less serious gastrointestinal side effects.

Sublingual immunotherapy (SLIT) is when food allergen extracts are formulated into drops that are placed under the tongue daily to help in a similar way to OIT. The advantage of SLIT is that the risk of reacting to doses is significantly lower compared to OIT. However, OIT is more effective in inducing desensitization compared to SLIT. Another type of immunotherapy that is in the early stages of development and involves an oral route is called oral mucosal immunotherapy (OMIT). Peanuts are the first food allergen to be used for this type of treatment. OMIT uses a specially formulated toothpaste that delivers small amounts of peanut protein to areas of the mouth and allows the immune system to interact with these tiny doses to induce desensitization.

Another route of administration for food allergen immunotherapy currently under investigation is called epicutaneous immunotherapy (EPIT). In this process, a food allergen is delivered to the skin through a patch. For young children, the patch is usually placed on the upper back, and it may be placed on the inner arm in older children. Multiple clinical trials have shown that EPIT can increase the dose needed to cause an allergic reaction by at least tenfold from baseline. Most participants in these studies reported mild skin reactions where the patch was located. Anaphylaxis was still reported in these studies.

Allergen Immunotherapy for Treating Allergic Rhinitis

Let's get back to Chelsea. She had heard about allergy shots from her neighbors, who had some good success, so she was interested in learning more about how they could help her. When I saw her, I performed a skin test, revealing that she was allergic to pollen, dust mites, and cats. She told me that she had already tried keeping her home as clean as possible and tried every OTC allergy medication that was available, but she was still suffering from symptoms, especially around cats. Chelsea asked me how allergy shots work.

Allergen immunotherapy (AIT) is the only treatment for allergic rhinitis that works on the underlying cause, which is the abnormal immune response to foreign substances like pollen and cat dander. Allergy shots are known as subcutaneous immunotherapy (SCIT) because the injections are given in the fatty tissue under the skin. There is also sublingual immunotherapy (SLIT) for environmental allergens in the form of tablets or allergy drops. I will not go into a lot of details about allergy drops because they are not approved by the FDA, but I will go over SLIT tablets because they are FDA-approved. Like OIT, SCIT involves increasing the doses of allergens until a maintenance dose is reached. Unlike OIT, the frequency of SCIT doses may be spaced out over time if the patient is maintaining clinical improvement.

Even though AIT has been used for over a hundred years, we do not fully understand how it works. There are several changes to the immune system that we know take place during AIT, including decreased mast cell activity, decreased allergen-specific IgE levels, increased allergen-specific IgG4 levels, and the generation of allergen-specific regulatory T and B cells that help suppress hypersensitivity reactions. We know that after several months of AIT, if someone is exposed to their allergen, their reactions are significantly reduced, but the mechanisms surrounding how this happens are not fully understood.

I often explain to my patients that AIT works in the same way that we get used to watching scary movies. As kids, we typically are afraid to watch scary movies. However, over time, we become numb or desensitized to the scary sounds and images on the screen. Another way to think about AIT is that we are making the immune system bored with the allergen through repeated exposure.

You may be wondering why usual exposure is not as effective as AIT. Can't Chelsea cause her immune system to become tolerant by living with a cat? It may be possible to get used to an animal, but that may come with a lot of unwanted symptoms, and it is not likely to work. AIT provides a controlled, low-dose exposure through either injection or under the tongue to engage with the immune system more directly. Usual exposure to allergens tends to activate already predetermined allergy pathways in the body.

There are various protocols for SCIT. They vary based on the number of injections per visit, number of visits per week, and how fast the maintenance dose is reached. While many protocols involve dosing once or twice a week, some offer an accelerated schedule known as rush or cluster immunotherapy. These schedules increase the risk of anaphylaxis, however. Once the buildup phase is completed, then doses are spaced out and given every two to four weeks for several years. The duration of SCIT is typically around five years so that the benefits obtained from this therapy last for several years after stopping it. However, it is not clear exactly how long this benefit may last. One of the most reliable indicators of the effectiveness of AIT is clinical history, and repeated allergy testing may or may not show a significant change compared to the previous allergy testing.

One of the potentially significant benefits of AIT is that it may delay or prevent the development of new allergen sensitivities. Roughly 20 percent of children who have allergic rhinitis develop asthma later in life. However, children who have completed AIT are less likely to develop asthma. In fact, a meta-analysis in 2017 including thirty-two studies estimated that the risk of developing asthma for children on AIT was reduced by as much as 60 percent. These benefits are likely due to reducing allergic inflammation during a time when a child's immune system is maturing.

AIT can be offered at any age, theoretically. However, children younger than five years old may not be able to verbalize any symptoms that may develop from the doses. SLIT may be a better option for younger children. On the other hand, there is really no age limit for AIT. While allergic inflammation tends to weaken in people sixty years and older, AIT may still be beneficial for some. During my allergy fellowship training, I remember taking care of a patient who was over one hundred years old and was still getting SCIT every four weeks!

While costs may vary for AIT, depending on insurance coverage, multiple studies have shown that AIT is cost-effective, especially if someone requires both nasal and inhaled medications. The economic benefits of AIT have been studied in Europe as well as the United States.

Adverse reactions to SCIT may occur. Injection site reactions are common and may include itching, redness, and swelling. The skin reactions may be tiny or large, but these symptoms do not significantly increase the risk of developing anaphylaxis due to an injection. Skin reactions are hard to predict. It is common for allergists to recommend taking an oral antihistamine one to three hours prior to an injection to help reduce the chances of developing a skin reaction. There is not much data regarding other potential preventive measures such as using topical steroids or cold packs, or dividing the dose between two arms. Some people may complain of increased symptoms for a couple of days after an injection is administered.

There is a risk of anaphylaxis after each dose of SCIT. However, the actual risk depends on several factors, including the amount of allergen administered, the type of allergen administered, and the dosing protocol. Most severe reactions to SCIT occur within the first thirty minutes of injection, so waiting in the office during that time will help identify and treat those severe reactions quickly. Deaths from SCIT have been reported, but this is very rare. It is estimated that fatal SCIT reactions occur once in 7.2 million injection visits. Most people who suffered fatal SCIT reactions had asthma that was uncontrolled, had previously experienced a systemic reaction, or received an erroneous dose. A class of medications called beta blockers, which are used to treat various cardiovascular diseases and anxiety, may make it difficult to treat anaphylaxis with epinephrine. Many allergists will ask patients to skip doses of their beta blocker medication when they are receiving SCIT doses.

I discussed the potential risks and benefits of SCIT with Chelsea and she seemed excited to start. My nurses asked for her informed consent and explained the process again for her before she got her first dose. Initially, the process felt slow and tedious. Chelsea struggled to consistently come every week, but she started to notice a significant improvement in her symptoms around cats after roughly six months. At that time, she could hold cats for several hours without feeling any severe symptoms. By twelve months, she took the leap and adopted a kitten, which she had dreamed about doing for most of her life. Chelsea was not completely free of symptoms, but she felt that she could manage her symptoms much better, and she did not need as much medication as she did prior to starting SCIT.

Unfortunately, while AIT is highly effective at improving symptoms and reducing medication burden, this therapy is not 100 percent effective. There are several potential reasons. People who are immunocompromised are less likely to respond well to AIT. People who are sensitized to multiple allergens are less likely to respond compared to those who are sensitized to only one allergen. A person with a prolonged history of allergic rhinitis before starting AIT is less likely to respond well than people who start earlier. There are studies that suggest that certain immune system signatures may be less likely to respond to AIT. For example, there is an association between people with a lower baseline ratio of allergen-specific IgE to total IgE and having a poorer response to AIT.

SCIT Versus SLIT for Treating Allergic Rhinitis

There are FDA-approved SLIT tablets for people who are sensitized to one allergen, including Oralair (five types of northern grass pollen), Grastek (timothy grass pollen), Ragwitek (short ragweed), and Odactra (dust mites). These are rapidly dissolving tablets that are held under the tongue for at least one minute or until completely dissolved. No food or drinks should be consumed for five minutes after the dose. The first dose is given under medical supervision and the patient is observed for signs of an allergic reaction for at least the first thirty minutes. The subsequent doses are taken once daily at home. If the tablet is for pollen allergy, then it is usually started three to four months before the pollen season starts. Dust mite tablets are usually taken year-round.

The most common side effects of SLIT tablets are oral itching, ear itching, sore throat, and swelling of the lips, tongue, or throat. A few cases of anaphylaxis have occurred from SLIT drops made at an allergist's office and not FDA-approved. Because of this risk, it is generally recommended to carry an epinephrine auto-injector. No fatal reactions have been reported due to SLIT tablets. Rare cases of eosinophilic esophagitis have been reported in people using SLIT.

Both SCIT and SLIT are effective treatments for allergic rhinitis. However, multiple studies have shown that SCIT is more effective than SLIT for reducing symptoms and medication use. But SLIT has fewer side effects than SCIT. SLIT is safe to take at home, but SCIT needs to be done in a clinic to monitor for severe reactions. Making the choice between SLIT and SCIT should include considering the potential risks and benefits of each therapy.

Venom Immunotherapy

AIT can be used to treat systemic allergic reactions to the venom from insects including bees, hornets, wasps, and fire ants. The treatment schedule is similar to AIT for environmental allergens. Chapter 12 discussed reasons for starting venom immunotherapy (VIT). While VIT can be highly effective at reducing the risk of developing anaphylaxis after subsequent stings, the degree of effectiveness varies between insect species. VIT is least effective for treating honeybee venom.

Severe symptoms may occur with VIT. However, if severe reactions occur multiple times, then a tryptase test may be needed to investigate possible mast cell disorders (see chapter 14). Most people will be on VIT for a minimum of three to five years to maximize protection and gain long-lasting benefits. However, some people may need to be on VIT indefinitely. Risk factors for requiring indefinite treatment include a life-threatening anaphylactic episode, a high like-lihood of recurrent stings due to either recreational or occupational activities, a honeybee allergy, or a history of a mast cell disorder.

TAKE-HOME POINTS

- Oral immunotherapy is not a cure for food allergies, but it may increase the amount of food allergen that can be tolerated if there is accidental ingestion.

- The risks and benefits of oral immunotherapy must be carefully considered before starting this procedure.

- The only disease-modifying treatment for many allergic diseases is allergen immunotherapy.

CHAPTER 17

Biologics

Anne adjusted her costume and looked around the bustling TV set. As an extra, she spent most of her time blending into the background, playing characters who rarely had lines but helped tell the story through their presence. It was not glamorous, but she enjoyed being a part of the TV industry. Her dream of being on-camera was unfortunately overshadowed by her relentless battle with severe asthma.

Over the past several years, she constantly struggled with difficulty breathing, wheezing, and chest tightness. Oftentimes, she could not work because she had a severe asthma attack and ended up in an emergency room receiving systemic steroids. She felt drained and discouraged constantly. One of her coworkers suggested that she see an allergist to help with her severe asthma.

When Anne met with me, I knew right away that we needed to make a change to her asthma regimen. It was not acceptable to be in the emergency room that frequently and she was struggling to do what she loved. After a lengthy conversation, we decided to start a biologic medication.

What Is a Biologic?

I highly recommend that you read through chapter 2 to get a better understanding of the immune system before reading the rest of this chapter. Otherwise, you may be asking a lot of questions and be left feeling confused.

Biologics are treatments derived from organic life such as microorganisms or animal cells. They are usually larger and more complex molecules than medications such as ibuprofen. Examples include vaccines, immunotherapy treatments for cancer, stem cell therapy, gene therapy, and skin grafts. In the context of allergic diseases, biologic medications usually come in the form of monoclonal antibodies (mAbs). These are antibodies that come from B cells produced in a lab; they come from one cell line that ends up creating an abundance of one antibody. Hence, the term *monoclonal*, meaning "coming from a single cell." A mAb is like a custom-designed key that fits perfectly into a specific lock. Traditional treatments are like traditional keys that fit several locks but do not always work perfectly. This is a targeted approach to treating diseases. These medications are typically given as an injection, usually through a subcutaneous route, meaning in the fatty tissue layer just beneath the skin.

There are mAbs approved for several allergic diseases, many of which we discussed in detail in part II of this book. In this chapter, I will go over the available biologics for each allergic disease that we discussed previously and use patient stories to help guide the discussion. If the disease has multiple medications available, then I will not name a specific biologic used in the story because I do not want to give the impression that I am endorsing a specific medication. I am trying to make sure that all these medications are discussed; if any seem applicable to you, then you should talk with your doctor about your potential options. Also, keep in mind that the mAb landscape is changing rapidly, so this information is subject to change. It is crucial to go over the potential benefits and risks of a medication with your doctor.

What Biologics Are Available for Allergic Diseases?

There are eight FDA-approved biologics available to treat various allergic diseases. While many of these medications are available to treat multiple diseases, not all eight are approved for the same ones. This section will name these medications and their specific targets.

Omalizumab (Xolair) was the first mAb approved (in 2003) to treat moderate-to-severe asthma. This mAb works by binding to a specific area of IgE that is freely available in the bloodstream, which prevents the IgE antibodies from attaching to the surface of mast cells and basophils at a receptor called FcεRI. Over time, there is a decrease in available FcεRI, so the mast cells and basophils become less sensitive to allergens. That means that these cells are less likely to activate and release inflammatory mediators such as histamine, leukotrienes, and prostaglandins. Xolair is given by subcutaneous injection every two to four weeks, depending on the disease that is being treated and the total number of IgE antibodies present.

Mepolizumab (Nucala) was approved in 2015 as the first mAb to bind directly to interleukin-5 (IL-5) to block its activity. This cytokine is responsible for promoting growth, activation, and survival of eosinophils. By blocking IL-5, this mAb helps reduce eosinophilic inflammation. Nucala is given every four weeks by subcutaneous injection. Reslizumab (Cinqair) is another IL-5 blocker that was FDA-approved in 2016, but this mAb is given by an intravenous infusion every two weeks (it is not available outside the US). Benralizumab (Fasenra) is another mAb that reduces eosinophilic inflammation and was approved in 2017, but the underlying mechanism is different. While Nucala and Cinqair bind directly to IL-5, Fasenra binds to IL-5 receptor alpha (IL-5Rα), which causes a phenomenon known as antibody-dependent cellular cytotoxicity (ADCC). This process involves antibodies binding to a target cell, triggering an immune response that kills the cell. In this case, Fasenra causes ADCC to fight against eosinophils, reducing eosinophilic inflammation. This mAb is a subcutaneous injection given every four weeks for the first three doses and then every eight weeks afterward.

Dupilumab (Dupixent) is a mAb that blocks IL-4 receptor alpha (IL-4Rα) and was initially approved in 2017 for moderate-to-severe eczema. Its target is a protein found in two receptors—IL-4 and IL-13. By targeting IL-4Rα, the signaling pathways for both IL-4 and IL-13 are reduced. This helps reduce eosinophilic inflammation, excess mucus production, IgE production, and airway hyperresponsiveness. Dupixent is a subcutaneous injection given every one to four weeks, depending on the disease being treated and the person's body weight.

Tezepelumab (Tezspire) targets thymic stromal lymphopoietin (TSLP) and was approved in 2021. This cytokine is released in response to environmental triggers such as allergens, viruses, and pollutants. TSLP activates multiple inflammatory pathways, which include IL-4, IL-5, and IL-13. Blocking TSLP helps reduce eosinophilic inflammation, allergic inflammation, and airway hyperresponsiveness. This mAb is a subcutaneous injection given every four weeks.

Another mAb approved in 2021 is tralokinumab (Adbry/Adtralza), which is approved for adults with moderate-to-severe eczema. In 2024, lebrikizumab (Ebglyss) was approved for people ages twelve and older who weigh at least 40 kg, for the treatment of moderate-to-severe eczema as well. These medications work slightly differently, but they both target IL-13 to reduce inflammation. This cytokine is involved in eczema because it promotes skin barrier dysfunction, increasing the risk of skin drying out. IL-13 recruits inflammatory cells to the skin, increases itching, and modifies the skin microbiome. Both Adbry/Adtralza and Ebglyss are initially given every two weeks for at least sixteen weeks and then may be spaced to every four weeks when the skin is well controlled.

These medications may take a couple of weeks to several months to start working effectively. There are multiple reasons why this may be the case. For example, since these therapies are highly targeted, it takes significantly more time for the body to adjust to the changes in the immune system. This process tends to take longer when someone has been experiencing severe symptoms for a long time. Also, each person's body may react differently to a mAb, so the time it takes to see results may vary. To address these issues, some of these medications require a "loading dose," which is a higher dose to start with, to reach therapeutic levels more quickly, and then the dose is decreased to a maintenance dose that is given consistently. If someone starts taking a mAb, it is best to wait at least four to six months before you can know the full benefits of the medication.

Biologics for Treating
Moderate-to-Severe Asthma

Let us get back to Anne for a moment. She was experiencing asthma attacks multiple times per year despite taking high-dose inhaled steroids. Her lung function test showed that she had obstructed airways. It was clear that she needed a change in her medication regimen, but when does someone need a biologic for asthma? A mAb is considered for people who have asthma symptoms despite taking standard controller medications, usually at a medium-to-high dose. Symptoms of asthma usually occur several days a week, requiring multiple doses of a rescue medication like salbutamol. The asthma symptoms may be severe enough to require an oral steroid, emergency room visit, and/or hospitalization. If this occurs two or more times in a year, then a mAb should be considered.

Anne had some testing done to help figure out the underlying molecular mechanism of her asthma, also known as her asthma endotype. In chapter 11, we discussed how there are different mechanisms for asthma. Testing may include a complete blood count, specifically looking for the total number of white blood cells called eosinophils. This test helps show whether eosinophilic inflammation is occurring. Another blood test measures the total IgE level, which helps determine whether allergic inflammation is present. Environmental allergy testing may be obtained to help establish whether allergic inflammation exists. This information helps doctors pick what may be the best mAb for you, because there are six FDA-approved biologics to treat moderate-to-severe asthma.

All the biologics mentioned previously are approved for asthma, but their effectiveness depends on their endotype. For example, if someone is allergic to pollen, dust mites, and pet dander and their total IgE level is high while their total eosinophils are normal, their underlying asthma is likely due to allergic inflammation. Xolair might be the best fit for that person. On the other hand, if there is no clear sign of whether the inflammation is primarily allergic or eosinophilic, then starting Tezspire may make more sense. There may be multiple choices for someone, especially if their underlying asthma is primarily due to eosinophilic inflammation.

After undergoing some testing and a rigorous discussion about the risks and benefits of the chosen mAb, Anne started her therapy in my clinic. Within a couple of months, she reported a tremendous amount of relief from her symptoms. What was most noticeable for her from the start was that she was not having daily asthma symptoms. She still relied on her daily controller medications, but instead of having an asthma attack five to six times per year, she was experiencing at most one attack per year. Her life quickly turned around and she was able to get back to being on a TV set.

Biologic for Treating Chronic Spontaneous Urticaria

Cheryl was always an optimist, but her life was turned upside down when she woke up one day with her face swollen and her chest covered in hives. She had no idea why this was happening. She tried taking Benadryl, but that was not working, so she went to urgent care and was prescribed a steroid pack. Her symptoms calmed down briefly, only to return with a vengeance. She came to see me after suffering for a month with urticaria and angioedema. I did some allergy testing and checked for any signs of thyroid disease or autoimmune disease, but all her tests came back normal. I prescribed high doses of a second-generation antihistamine and Pepcid (famotidine) to try to calm her hives, but that did not help either.

We discussed Xolair as a choice for her. This mAb was approved in 2014 for the treatment of chronic spontaneous urticaria for people twelve years and older when antihistamine therapy does not work, especially if medications had been taken for six or more weeks. In a meta-analysis of seven randomized clinical trials with over 1,300 people, 36 percent reported a complete response to Xolair. While this mAb can be a highly effective treatment for urticaria, it is difficult to know when to stop Xolair because urticaria can resolve on its own, but people may relapse after stopping Xolair.

While Xolair is generally well tolerated, the FDA put a black box warning on the medication in 2007 because of the risk of developing anaphylaxis. Anaphylaxis has developed in one to two per 1,000 people receiving Xolair. It is not clear why these reactions occur. Anaphylaxis can occur after any dose and usually happens within the first two hours after an injection. This is why it is recommended that Xolair be given in a clinic and people be monitored closely after each injection.

Initially, there was some concern about the possibility of Xolair increasing the risk of developing cancer. However, in 2012, there was a systematic review of thirty-two clinical trials that identified 14 cases of cancer in 4,254 people who were treated with Xolair compared to 11 cases of cancer in 3,178 people who were treated with a placebo. This means that the rate of cancer was similar regardless of whether Xolair was given. There were no clear patterns in the characteristics of these cancers, so it is unlikely that Xolair increases the risk of developing cancer. There have also been concerns raised about the potential increased risk of developing cardiovascular disease. In 2014, the FDA released a statement that, based on an analysis of twenty-five randomized clinical trials, there did not appear to be a significantly increased risk. It is also difficult to determine whether Xolair does increase the risk of cardiovascular disease because the patients studied typically had more severe asthma than the control groups. Severe asthma can be a risk factor for cardiovascular disease, so this may have skewed the results.

Cheryl decided to start Xolair, but it did not work right away. She needed two doses before she began to see significant improvements. After four months of therapy, she was able to reduce her antihistamine use to one pill a day, and she was not having difficulty with sleeping or intense itching. She was able to get back to her life and not have to deal with the constant dread of when her hives would return.

Biologics to Treat Chronic Rhinosinusitis with Nasal Polyps

Jeff has struggled with nasal polyps for most of his adult life. He could not remember the last time he had a sense of smell. Life felt dull and gray. He was frustrated that he could not get relief despite using a neti pot every day and taking nasal sprays. He even had two sinus surgeries to remove polyps and fix his deviated nasal septum, but he constantly felt congested. At the same time, he had asthma that required daily medication to keep his symptoms under control. Jeff decided finally to speak to an allergist about starting a biologic medication because he was desperate to find relief.

Treating CRS with nasal polyps using biologics is a relatively new strategy. In 2019, Dupixent was FDA-approved to treat it and can be given to people as young as twelve years old. However, if a child has nasal polyps, then testing needs to be done to rule out cystic fibrosis, since there is a strong association between these conditions in children. Nucala and Xolair are also approved to treat CRS with nasal polyps. Biologics are not approved for CRS when there are no nasal polyps. A mAb is usually considered for people with CRS with nasal polyps when their symptoms return despite their having had sinus surgery. Some people may start with a biologic if they cannot get sinus surgery or have severe asthma. These biologics have all been able to improve quality of life through reducing nasal congestion and nasal polyps as well as improving sense of smell.

For Jeff, his choice to start a biologic led to incremental improvements in his sense of smell over three months. While his sinus pain never completely went away, his symptoms became manageable. He was very pleased with the improvements in his asthma symptoms, which felt like an unexpected side benefit. He became more hopeful for the future now that his polyps were gone.

Biologics to Treat Food Allergies

Ariana had been allergic to peanuts and tree nuts for as long as she could remember. Her mother told her that, as a baby, she had hives all over her body after eating peanut butter. For most of her childhood, she was able to cope with avoiding nuts and rarely had any reactions. Now in her thirties, she started to struggle. For the past couple of years, she had experienced anaphylaxis multiple times. She felt that she was doing everything right—reading food labels carefully, communicating her food allergies at restaurants, and avoiding cross-contamination. Ariana believed that her immune system was becoming more sensitive. Over time, she became anxious and avoided eating out at restaurants or going to social events.

Ariana was losing hope that she could feel like herself again until she heard about Xolair being approved to treat food allergies. In February 2024, the FDA approved Xolair for IgE-mediated food allergy for people as young as one year or older to reduce the risk of anaphylaxis that may occur with accidental exposure to one or more foods. This approval was based on a clinical trial called Omalizumab as Monotherapy and as Adjunct Therapy to Multi-Allergen Oral Immunotherapy in Food Allergic Children and Adults, which I know is a mouthful, but it is referred to as the OUtMATCH trial. There were 177 children and adolescents in the trial allergic to peanuts and at least two other foods who were randomized to receive

Xolair or a placebo every two to four weeks, based on their body weight and total blood IgE levels. The participants did not know what therapy they were receiving, nor did the people administering the therapy, to help reduce the chance of bias in the study. After sixteen weeks of therapy, they were given oral food challenges and 67 percent of the participants who were taking Xolair were able to consume 600 mg of peanut protein without any symptoms compared to only 7 percent in the placebo group. Similar results were shown for most other foods tested, including eggs and cow's milk. Only 41 percent of participants allergic to cashew could tolerate at least 1,000 mg of protein when given Xolair.

There are multiple phases of the OUtMATCH trial still underway to answer questions such as comparing Xolair to oral immunotherapy (see chapter 16) and what happens when Xolair is discontinued after one year. Ariana understood that she would not be able to eat her food allergens freely, but she was hopeful that her reactions would be either minimal or eliminated. She started Xolair and has so far been doing well.

Food is implicated as a trigger for symptoms of eosinophilic esophagitis (EOE). In May 2022, the FDA approved Dupixent to treat EOE and in January 2024 it became available to children as young as one year and weighing at least 15 kg (it is also approved in the EU, Canada and Australia). This medication is given every two weeks if someone weighs less than 40 kg. For people who are 40 kg or more, the medication is given once weekly. This approval was based on multiple studies showing significant improvement in the number of eosinophils found through esophageal biopsy and in difficulty swallowing (i.e., dysphagia) when taking Dupixent compared to a placebo. The full role of Dupixent in treating EOE is still under active investigation, but this biologic holds tremendous potential for people who struggle with EOE despite elimination diets and swallowed steroids.

Biologics to Treat Eczema

Do you remember Eric, who I talked about in chapter 8? He was the child who had severe eczema that was difficult to control despite multiple topical medications. Trying to relieve his skin condition was taking a severe toll on his parents. Because he was three years old, the only mAb available to him was Dupixent. Multiple clinical trials have investigated the safety and efficacy of Dupixent for treating moderate-to-severe eczema in people ages six months and older. The clinical trial that led to FDA approval for infants and toddlers to use it for eczema reported that 28 percent of study participants taking Dupixent had clear or near clear skin compared to 4 percent with placebo, while 53 percent had at least 75 percent improvement in their skin compared to 11 percent with placebo.

Common side effects reported with Dupixent for treating eczema include injection site reactions, red eyes (conjunctivitis), and facial redness. It is unclear why people may develop red eyes when starting Dupixent. Oftentimes, this symptom appears in the first few weeks or months of therapy and then resolves with continued treatment. If this becomes persistent, then an ophthalmologist may be needed to address these concerns. It is also unclear why some people develop a rash on their face and/or neck while taking Dupixent. Various topical medications have been tried to treat this side effect and have shown variable results.

While Eric did remarkably well after Dupixent was started, he developed red eyes roughly six months after starting this therapy. I sent him to an ophthalmologist, who did not find any vision problems and prescribed eye drops for him. After approximately six weeks, his eyes returned to normal, and his skin continued to be almost clear.

Considerations When
Starting a Biologic

I have been asked many questions surrounding biologic medications and I want to finish this chapter by providing answers to some of the most frequently asked ones. First, a mAb does not necessarily fix the problem nor is it a cure. These medications are highly effective at turning off one portion of the immune system, but there could be several other inflammatory pathways still active. Think of a mAb like a patch for a leaky pipe. The patch may target the leak directly, but it may not fully address the underlying problem, which could be a crack further down the pipe.

Access to these medications can be difficult because mAbs can be very expensive. One study published in 2018 looked at the monoclonal antibodies approved by the FDA from 1997 to 2016 and estimated that the average annual cost was over $96,000. However, this study included cancer treatments, which made the cost much higher than it would be otherwise. The annual cost of Cinqair was $40,381 and Xolair was $30,693. These medications are very expensive for many reasons. The research and testing needed to develop a safe and effective mAb is costly and the biomanufacturing process to produce a mAb is very resource-intensive. Whether the high cost of biologics for both patients and insurance companies/healthcare providers outweighs the potential costs incurred by severe disease is still under investigation.

One of the biggest concerns I hear from my patients is about the potential long-term side effects of monoclonal antibodies, especially for children. Xolair has been approved by the FDA since 2003, so there is more long-term safety data with that medication, which we discussed earlier in the chapter. However, most of the other biologics have only been around for ten years or less. Fortunately, these medications are constantly scrutinized, and safety data continues to be reported. If you are considering a mAb for yourself or your child, it may feel like a leap of faith. It is normal to feel nervous about starting a medication that can alter your immune system.

Giving your informed consent involves weighing the potential benefits and risks of an intervention versus the benefits and risks of an alternative. As an example, some people with severe asthma become dependent on taking oral steroids every day to improve their asthma symptoms and reduce the risk of experiencing a severe asthma attack. Systemic steroids can carry some serious risks, including immunosuppression, osteoporosis, and diabetes. A mAb may have the ability to reduce their overall exposure to systemic steroids. However, the potential risks may outweigh the benefits in certain situations. As an example, the safety of biologics during pregnancy is not well established. A careful discussion with your specialists is needed to weigh the potential risks and benefits not only for the mother but also for the developing fetus.

Another challenge with mAbs is that it is difficult to know if or when these medications can be stopped. These medications are also not meant to be taken seasonally. If the biologic is stopped, symptoms are likely to return because the biologics do not cure the disease but only temporarily reduce the symptoms. Some potential exceptions to this include chronic spontaneous urticaria and severe eczema in children. These are conditions that may be outgrown naturally.

It is astonishing how much progress we have made in the past twenty years to help treat severe allergic diseases. Multiple monoclonal antibodies have helped millions of people who had been suffering when there were not many good options previously. I hope that access to these amazing medications will improve in the future and that we will continue to improve our understanding of how biologics can help people living with these ailments.

TAKE-HOME POINTS

- There are eight monoclonal antibodies available to treat various allergic diseases.

- Treatment with a monoclonal antibody is usually indefinite.

- While these treatments can be highly effective, access to monoclonal antibodies may be limited, and they are almost always expensive.

CHAPTER 18

Future Directions

The management of allergic diseases is on the brink of transformation. There have been significant advances in immunology, precision medicine, biotechnology, and artificial intelligence. Traditional methods of testing and treatment will give way to more predictive and preventive approaches in the future. There are newer testing methods and treatment strategies under active investigation for many of the diseases that have been discussed throughout this book. As research continues to uncover the underlying mechanisms of allergic diseases, the next generation of advancements aims not only to manage symptoms but to modify the immune system itself, potentially changing the landscape of allergy care forever. This final chapter will discuss some of the newest developments and where we may be heading for many of the allergic diseases that we've discussed here.

Keep in mind that because medical advancements are appearing rapidly, some of what is discussed in this chapter may be currently available or scrapped because it did not end up working or the company developing the therapy did not want to spend more money. When I was combing the medical literature for what is currently being investigated by scientists, I frequently found review articles that discussed promising treatments, only to discover that they had been discontinued shortly thereafter. The information here is meant to show you that a lot of work is happening to try and manage these diseases more effectively. Also, if you are interested in learning more about newer treatments, check out clinicaltrials.gov. You may even want to be a part of a clinical trial to not only help yourself but also help the global community develop new treatments.

Allergic Rhinitis

For allergic rhinitis treatment to be successful, accurate testing is key. As discussed in chapter 4, there are skin tests and blood tests that measure for immunoglobulin E (IgE), which can potentially cause an allergic reaction to a substance. Component-resolved diagnostics (CRD) has been emerging as a blood test that may improve the accuracy of allergy testing. This is a modern approach that identifies specific allergenic proteins rather than whole allergen extracts. In other words, this testing looks at a component of an allergen rather than the entire part to help determine whether there is a risk of a serious allergic reaction. I believe that CRD will become more popular in the future as our understanding of allergens improves.

While subcutaneous immunotherapy and sublingual immunotherapy have been successful in treating allergic rhinitis, there have been alternative routes of administration under investigation to improve the effectiveness of immunotherapy. Intralymphatic immunotherapy (ILIT) is currently available in the United States but is not approved by the FDA. In this technique, FDA-approved allergen extracts are injected with ultrasound guidance into the inguinal lymph nodes, which are located near the groin. Usually, there are three sets of injections that are administered four weeks apart for a total treatment time of eight weeks. However, this requires specialized training to give precise injections close to the lymph node. Nasal sprays and topical therapies using patches have also been investigated.

While side effects have been relatively mild, the symptoms have been bothersome enough that roughly 10 percent of study participants have dropped out due to discomfort.

Since the late 1980s, scientists have been trying to clone environmental allergens to be able to alter them in ways that they can become more standardized and modified to improve the immune response. These proteins are often referred to as recombinant allergens and could theoretically be produced in a large amount relatively quickly. The first clinical trial using recombinant allergens took place in the early 2000s. So far, the data has not shown that recombinant allergens are superior to classical extracts currently being used for immunotherapy. This option could potentially be viable in the future as we become more aware of how to map a patient's individual allergen profile.

Allergen vaccines are under development. Researchers have investigated mRNA and DNA vaccines for environmental allergens, but there have been no studies that have reached a phase III clinical trial yet. There is a newer type of vaccine that uses viruslike particles (VLPs) to help treat food allergies. VLPs are designed to look like viruses, but they do not cause an infection. Instead, they introduce parts of the allergen to help shift the immune response toward tolerating the allergen.

Sinusitis

There are some recent developments in treating chronic sinusitis with or without nasal polyps. For example, there are implants containing steroids that are placed in the sinus cavities, where they slowly release the medicine over thirty to ninety days, depending on the device, which may help reduce the inflammation in these areas. The two FDA-approved implants are Propel (mometasone furoate) and Sinuva (mometasone furoate). Precision medicine is increasingly being studied to better understand and manage chronic sinusitis by tailoring treatments to a person's specific immune profile. Researchers are working to characterize the underlying mechanisms of this disease, which will help develop newer, more targeted approaches.

Food Allergy

Unfortunately, we have seen a significant rise in the number of people affected by food allergies over the past thirty years. However, this has provided an opportunity for a significant influx of interest in research. Much work is needed to gain a better understanding of why food allergies have become increasingly more common. While multiple epidemiological studies are ongoing, there are multiple diagnostic and therapeutic interventions under active investigation that I am personally excited about. I could write an entire chapter on food allergy alone, but I will provide the highlights in this section.

One of the greatest challenges in food allergy is providing a safe, yet accurate diagnosis. The testing currently available has relatively low specificity, meaning that the tests are not very good at correctly identifying who does not have food allergy. In other words, some people are potentially carrying a diagnosis of food allergy but are not actually allergic. I have seen many patients in my clinic who have been labeled with multiple food allergies but, with careful testing, turn out to have fewer allergies than they initially thought.

The basophil activation test (BAT) measures the expression of markers such as CD63 and CD203c that are on the surface of basophils that are stimulated by the allergen in question. BAT appears to have a higher specificity compared to skin or IgE blood testing. This test may help distinguish people who are truly allergic from those who are sensitized to the food but are able to eat it. The problem with BAT currently is that it is not widely available because it requires specialized techniques such as flow cytometry, needs fresh blood samples, and the protocols are not completely standardized.

The interpretation of the BAT may be inconsistent. For now, this tool is considered more for research purposes.

Machine learning and diagnostic algorithms are being researched to help improve diagnostic accuracy. For example, there is the Nut Co-reactivity-Acquiring Knowledge for Elimination Recommendations (NUT CRACKER) diagnostic algorithm for cashew allergy that combines a cashew skin test with BAT and the cashew allergen component Ana o 3 to reduce by 72 percent the number of oral food challenges needed to identify who is allergic to cashews. There is also a predictive tool available online for peanut allergy that uses the peanut skin test, BAT, and peanut allergen component Ara h 2 to help predict the potential severity of an allergic reaction.

There is technology in development to help detect allergens in food. There is a product called the Allergy Amulet that uses sensors with trillions of tiny cavities that bind to specific allergens. If the food allergen is present, a unique electric signal is sent to alert the user. The test takes approximately one minute to complete. This device is currently able to detect peanuts (at 1 mg/100 g food), soy (at 10 mg/100 g food), and gluten (at 2 mg/100 g food), but there are plans to include the top nine most common food allergens.

While chapter 16 discussed various immunotherapy strategies such as oral immunotherapy, epicutaneous immunotherapy, and oral mucosal immunotherapy, there are several other therapeutic strategies under investigation. An Australian company called Aravax is currently administering a phase II clinical trial on their product PVX108. This is a treatment for peanut allergy that theoretically works similarly to other immunotherapy methods, but it consists of intradermal injections of peanut peptides instead of whole peanut protein. This is being administered once a month to help reduce the risk of anaphylaxis if there is accidental ingestion.

Vaccines are under development for treating food allergies. VLP vaccines produce an immune response that helps shift antibody production toward the more tolerant IgG antibodies. Another vaccine strategy under investigation is an mRNA platform. Scientists have developed tiny fat substances called lipid nanoparticles that specifically target liver cells to unload an mRNA strand that instructs the liver to produce the Ara h 2 portion of the peanut protein. In mice, this technology has been shown to alter the immune system's response toward promoting tolerance to peanuts.

A cancer medication called acalabrutinib used to treat lymphoma may be used to treat food allergy. This medication inhibits an enzyme called Bruton's tyrosine kinase (BTK), which is involved in sending signals to B cells that allow them to mature and produce antibodies that may be necessary for creating an allergic reaction. Recently, acalabrutinib was studied in ten adults allergic to peanuts and they were able to tolerate a 32- to 217-fold higher amount of peanut protein than their baseline.

There is great interest in researching therapeutics related to human gut microbiome. The gut bacterial environment during the twenty-first century has significantly shifted because of overuse of antibiotics, low-fiber diets, formula feeding, early antacid use, and cesarean births. These may be risk factors for developing food allergies. There are clinical trials investigating whether food allergies can be treated using fecal transplantation. Probiotics are also under active investigation.

Another interesting approach to treating food allergies is to use multiple monoclonal antibodies at the same time. There is a monoclonal antibody called linvoseltamab that is being developed to treat a cancer called multiple myeloma. The cells affected in multiple myeloma are plasma cells that produce antibodies. Linvoseltamab works by connecting multiple myeloma cells with T cells to promote T cells to kill these cancer cells. This medication broadly removes plasma cells that are consistently producing antibodies. Dupilumab (Dupixent) helps prevent B cells from producing IgE antibodies. Therefore, using linvoseltamab and dupilumab in combination would help prevent allergic reactions, which was shown in a study involving mice. Currently, a phase I study in humans is underway to determine whether this novel approach could be safe.

Eczema

The foundation of eczema therapy is to moisturize the skin well to help maintain a good skin barrier. There are numerous moisturizers and topical medications under development and many that have been recently FDA-approved. For example, there is a cream called asivatrep that blocks the transient receptor potential vanilloid subfamily V member 1 (TRPV1), which is found in the skin and is involved in the sensation of itch and regulating inflammation. Although asivatrep has not been FDA-approved as of the writing of this book, the results so far seem positive in multiple clinical trials. In December 2024, tapinarof (Vtama) 1 percent cream was FDA-approved to treat eczema for individuals two years and older, though it is not yet available outside the US. This medication binds to the aryl hydrocarbon receptor (AhR), which regulates cytokine and skin barrier protein expression as well as antioxidant activity. What is positive about these medications is that they are both not steroids.

If you remember, in chapter 8, we discussed how the bacteria on the skin of people living with eczema are altered. This is often referred to as cutaneous dysbiosis. A bacterium called *Roseomonas mucosa* that is found in people who do not have eczema has been used in clinical trials as a topical therapy. The data from those clinical trials showed mixed results in their effectiveness. *Staphylococcus hominis* A9 is another bacterium on healthy skin that has been found to be effective in a small clinical trial of fifty-four adults who had eczema that contained the harmful bacteria *Staphylococcus aureus*. There is a bacterium that can produce nitric oxide, called *Nitrosomonas eutropha*, which has anti-inflammatory properties. Three clinical trials are underway investigating whether *N. eutropha* is beneficial.

As our understanding of eczema grows, so also do the potential targets for treatment. For example, a protein called OX40L is found on antigen-presenting cells and binds to a protein called OX40 found on activated T cells; it plays a crucial role in causing the inflammation seen in eczema. There is a monoclonal antibody called rocatinlimab that targets OX40, while there is another antibody called amlite-limab that targets OX40L. Both medications are potentially promising options for treating eczema in the future.

Contact Dermatitis

Much of the research into contact dermatitis is focused on understanding the underlying mechanisms of how contact dermatitis develops. This skin disease can be difficult to diagnose because the rash does not have specific clinical characteristics that distinguish it from other similar skin diseases. The general principles of the patch test have remained mostly unchanged since 1894 when it was introduced by German dermatologist Josef Jadassohn (1863–1936). This test can be costly, time consuming, and resource-intensive, so many people do not have access to patch testing. Therefore, we need a better understanding of contact dermatitis so that we can develop more efficient testing in the future.

Urticaria and Angioedema

Multiple BTK blockers are under development for the treatment of chronic spontaneous urticaria (CSU). The medication in this category that is furthest along is remibrutinib, which is an oral medication. There are two phase III clinical trials, called REMIX-1 and REMIX-2, that were randomized, double-blind, placebo-controlled clinical trials consisting of over 800 adults with CSU. According to the press release by the pharmaceutical manufacturer Novartis, significant improvements in their symptoms occurred within the first twelve weeks of treatment and were sustained through fifty-two weeks of treatment. Almost half the patients were completely free of hives and itching at week 52 in the study. This data looks promising, and Novartis is working on filing for FDA approval at the time of writing this book.

The company Celldex recently completed a phase II clinical trial for its medication called barzolvolimab. This is a monoclonal antibody that blocks the activation of a protein called KIT, which is important for the maturation and survival of mast cells. There are now two phase III clinical trials underway, called EMBARQ-CSU1 and EMBARQ-CSU2. This medication may be beneficial for people who suffer from mast cell disorders. Another anti-KIT antibody called briquilimab is being studied in adults with CSU who are still symptomatic despite treatment with omalizumab (Xolair) or who cannot tolerate this medication.

While hereditary angioedema (HAE) is a rare disease, there are some potential new treatments on the horizon. There is a monoclonal antibody called garadacimab that blocks factor XIIa, which is one of the molecules responsible for the swelling attacks that occur due to HAE. Results from a recent phase III clinical trial appear to be promising. Gene editing has been studied to treat HAE, and a phase III study of the NTLA-2002 CRISPR gene editing treatment was recently started. This could become the first one-time treatment for HAE to prevent swelling attacks by inactivating the kallikrein B1 gene that encodes prekallikrein. This is a precursor protein to kallikrein that ends up causing the release of bradykinin, the culprit peptide responsible for causing fluid to leak from blood vessels.

Asthma

As our understanding of asthma evolves, researchers are developing not only new treatments but also strategies to help prevent the development of asthma. One of the substances involved in triggering allergic inflammation in asthma is IgE. Researchers started to wonder whether blocking IgE with Xolair early in life could prevent asthma. They started a first-of-its-kind clinical trial called Preventing Asthma in High Risk Kids (PARK). When I was a clinical fellow in allergy/immunology, I helped recruit study participants for the PARK study. They enrolled 200 kids from thirteen study locations throughout the United States who were two to three years old and had a history of two to four wheezing episodes in the past year, positive allergy testing to an environmental allergen, and a first-degree relative with a history of asthma or allergy. These children were considered at high risk for developing asthma. The PARK study was randomized, double-blind, and placebo controlled, so the study participants got either Xolair or a placebo and no one involved in receiving or administering the medication knew what was given, to reduce bias in the study. These children received the study drug for two years and then were observed for two years off the medication to see whether any participants developed asthma. At the time of writing this book, the results have not been published, but I am excited to see what comes from this incredibly labor-intensive study. To give you some perspective, it took over ten years for the FDA to approve the use of Xolair for children as young as two years old. Regardless of the results, the PARK study will provide us with valuable information.

Scientists have developed a bread that contains a variation of brewer's yeast usually used to make beer, called *Saccharomyces cerevisiae* UFMG A-905, which acts as a probiotic. In mice who were fed this probiotic bread, there were significant reductions in signs of airway inflammation such as eosinophils and concentrations of pro-inflammatory IL-5 and IL-13. This could potentially be a viable method for reducing asthma symptoms, but human clinical trials are needed to understand its full benefit.

In chapter 11, we discussed how asthma is not necessarily one disease because there are multiple underlying mechanisms, or endotypes, that can cause it. Our understanding of asthma endotypes has evolved rapidly in the past couple of decades. In 2025, a team of researchers developed a nasal swab that can identify the asthma endotype without needing any blood tests, skin tests, or pulmonary function tests. The nasal swab is like a COVID-19 swab, but it does not require the swab to reach the back of the nose to get a proper sample. This kind of breakthrough will help scientists be able to study asthma more effectively.

Recently, researchers discovered a protein called Piezo1 that prevents a type of immune cell, called Type 2 innate lymphoid cell (ILC2), from causing inflammation in the lungs that may result in asthma symptoms. If Piezo1 is absent, then more airway inflammation occurs. However, a drug called Yoda1 was able to increase the levels of Piezo1 to reduce the activity of ILC2s, thereby reducing inflammation in the lungs of mice. The small molecule Yoda1 was named after the fictional character Yoda in *Star Wars*, and this molecule was modified, which produced an antagonist molecule to Yoda1 called Dooku1, which was named after the *Star Wars* character Count Dooku. Yoda1 needs further studies to unlock its potential therapeutic benefit for asthma.

There are multiple medications under development for treating asthma. One of the challenges of biologic medications is that they need to be administered frequently, often every two to four weeks. There is a monoclonal antibody called depemokimab that blocks the pro-inflammatory effects of IL-5 and is ultra-long-acting. This medication can be given once every six months. A phase III clinical trial was published in 2024 that showed a significant reduction in the rate of severe asthma attacks in a year when close to 800 adults with eosinophilic asthma were given depemokimab compared to a placebo.

There is also an existing biologic medication that has shown promise in treating severe asthma attacks and potentially reducing the need for systemic steroids. Benralizumab (Fasenra) was used in a clinical trial to treat patients with severe asthma attacks and compared them to patients who were treated with the oral steroid prednisone. Those who were given benralizumab were significantly less likely to develop a treatment failure than those who were given prednisone.

While tezepelumab (Tezspire) is the first monoclonal antibody that blocks TSLP to treat severe asthma, there was another TSLP inhibitor in development called ecleralimab that was given as an inhaler. Unfortunately, the manufacturer stopped developing this medication.

Prior to studying asthma during my fellowship, I did not realize that many inhalers used to treat asthma have the potential to emit significant amounts of greenhouse gases, which can contribute to warming the planet. The hydrofluorocarbon propellants used in the pressurized metered-dose inhalers have a significantly higher global warming potential than the commonly known greenhouse gas carbon dioxide. While calls have been made to switch people to dry powder inhalers, pharmaceutical companies are working on developing inhalers with propellants that have a lower environmental impact. This will become increasingly more important since more people are being diagnosed with asthma globally.

Anaphylaxis

Significant advancements in treating anaphylaxis have happened recently. The first needle-free device containing epinephrine to treat anaphylaxis, Neffy, was approved by the FDA in August 2024 (it is also now available in the UK, Canada and the EU). This approval was initially for people who weighed at least 30 kg, but in March 2025, Neffy came out with a lower dose that was approved in the US for children weighing at least 15 kg. Now other needle-free epinephrine options are under development and may be available soon. A film containing the medication epinephrine, called Anaphylm, is placed under the tongue to treat anaphylaxis. This may be available as early as 2026.

A second nasal spray containing epinephrine is under investigation as well. It is called NDS1C in studies and it is two sprays for a single dose. It is unclear when this medication may be available. There is another device that contains an epinephrine powder called OX640 that is delivered nasally, but several human clinical trials still need to be completed before it is potentially released.

Recently, researchers explored new ways to use nanoparticles to help improve delivery of treatments. They used nanoparticles to target mast cells to block anaphylaxis in mice by coating the nanoparticles with two types of antibodies that would shut down the mast cells. Intravenous injections of these nanoparticles led to almost complete prevention of anaphylaxis with no significant side effects. It will take time to use these nanoparticles on humans, but this is an exciting development that may have applications for other allergic diseases.

Medication Allergies

As discussed in chapter 13, penicillin allergy is the most reported drug allergy in the United States, but only a small portion of people who think they are allergic to penicillin are actually allergic to this medication. A concerted effort is being made by researchers to improve the diagnostic accuracy of penicillin allergies. Various decision tools have been developed to help primary care physicians and allergists make more accurate diagnoses. The work that needs to be done to help safely and accurately remove penicillin allergies from people's medical records requires help not only from allergists but also from general practitioners, nurses, pharmacists, nurse practitioners, physician associates, nursing students, medical students, and pharmacy students. Hospitals will need to implement new policies and procedures that prioritize accurate drug allergy labeling to help improve patient outcomes.

Mast Cell Disorders

One of the major challenges with treating mast cell activation syndrome (MCAS) is that this clinical entity is extremely complex and not well defined. However, I believe that there is hope for better treatments for MCAS because our understanding of mast cell physiology has significantly improved over the past few decades. For example, there is a receptor called the Mas-related G protein-coupled receptor X2 (MRGPRX2) that is present on mast cells in the skin. Multiple studies have shown that MRGPRX2 is involved in mast cell activation for diseases such as eczema, chronic urticaria, asthma, and drug allergies. This receptor does not require IgE antibodies for activation. A drug called EP262, which blocks the effects of MRG-PRX2, is currently in clinical trials for chronic spontaneous urticaria. If the clinical trials report positive results, then this may be a potential MCAS treatment.

Another potential target under investigation is sialic acid-binding immunoglobulin-like lectins (Siglecs) that are found on eosinophils, mast cells, and basophils. These receptors recognize sialic acids, which are sugars that are found on the surface of human cells, so Siglecs help distinguish between "self" and "non-self," preventing excessive immune system activation. A monoclonal antibody called lirentelimab targets Siglec-8, which can inhibit mast cell activation. Unfortunately, in a phase II clinical trial for treating chronic spontaneous urticaria and eczema, this medication did not reach its primary goal, so it was not developed further. However, a similar molecule called AK006 is still under investigation; it targets Siglec-6, which is found on mast cells and basophils.

For people who have MCAS due to elevated mast cell burden such as systemic mastocytosis, a strategy may be to deplete their mast cell counts completely. There is a chemotherapy drug called cladribine that can reduce episodes of anaphylaxis for people who have systemic mastocytosis. However, this medication can cause significant immunosuppression, so it cannot be considered the first-line therapy for monoclonal mast cell activation syndrome or idiopathic MCAS.

Idiopathic MCAS is in desperate need of research into its underlying mechanisms and for more accurate testing that is more easily accessible. Large randomized, double-blind, placebo-controlled studies investigating current treatments such as high-dose H1-antihistamines are needed to clarify their effectiveness. More education and advocacy are needed to help raise awareness of these issues. I had never heard of these disorders in medical school, but I am hopeful that more people are becoming aware of them.

Final Thoughts

The burden of allergic diseases continues to grow. These conditions used to be dismissed as minor nuisances or were highly misunderstood, but they are now considered to be a significant public health challenge as millions of people are now affected. Even if these issues do not directly impact you, I am certain that you know at least one other person who faces significant challenges with at least one ailment that was discussed in this book.

Science and medicine have been evolving at a fast pace since the early twentieth century, but the field of allergy has advanced even more quickly. With each breakthrough in our understanding of allergic diseases, the future holds promise for better treatments and possibly cures. I hope the information in this book has helped empower you to have a deeper understanding of these conditions, their impact on individuals and communities, and their scientific progress shaping the future of allergy care. Knowledge is a powerful tool that we can use to advocate for better awareness, treatment, and support for those living with allergic diseases.

International Resources

Allergy UK – A leading British charity providing information, support, and advocacy for people living with allergic disease. It also works to raise awareness and influence public policy around allergy care in the UK.

Anaphylaxis UK – A UK-based charity focused on supporting individuals at risk of severe allergic reactions. It offers guidance on allergy management, adrenaline auto-injectors, and emergency preparedness for schools and workplaces.

Asthma + Lung UK – The UK's major charity dedicated to improving the lives of people with asthma and other lung conditions through education, research funding, and policy advocacy.

British Society for Allergy & Clinical Immunology (BSACI) – The UK's professional body representing allergists, immunologists, and related clinicians. BSACI develops clinical guidelines and promotes education and research in allergy and immunology.

European Academy of Allergy & Clinical Immunology (EAACI) – A Europe-wide professional organisation advancing research, education, and clinical practice in allergy and immunology, with thousands of members from across the continent.

World Allergy Organization (WAO) – A global federation of national and regional allergy societies that promotes the exchange of scientific knowledge, education, and training in allergy and clinical immunology worldwide.

Australasian Society of Clinical Immunology and Allergy (ASCIA) – The peak professional body for allergy and immunology specialists in Australia and New Zealand, providing educational resources and clinical guidelines for healthcare professionals and patients.

Canadian Society of Allergy and Clinical Immunology (CSACI) – Canada's national professional organisation for allergists and clinical immunologists, supporting research, education, and advocacy in allergic and immune-mediated diseases.

Acknowledgments

I never thought I would be able to write a book, but a village of people supported me along the way to help make this dream a reality. I want to thank so many people who helped me get here. Their encouragement, expertise, and belief in my message gave me the confidence to keep going, even when the process felt overwhelming. First, I want to explain to you how this book came about.

In June 2024, I got a message on my desk at my office in Naperville from Susan Roxborough, who is a senior editor at Clarkson Potter. She had been following my social media content for a while and suggested that I write a book about allergy and immunology. She explained to me that she was struggling with understanding some immunologic issues that were affecting her family and that I could provide a helpful resource for many people. Susan connected me with my literary agents, Mia Vitale and Sarah Passick at Park & Fine (now Park, Fine & Brower). They were instrumental in helping me with my book proposal and connecting me with Plume. Mia and Sarah have been amazing to me!

Karen Tang is an ob-gyn who I have been friends with for several years through our work on social media together. She was a mentor for me during the entire process of navigating literary agents, publishers, and book writing. I really appreciate all her time and help throughout the years. She always made herself available to me through calls or texting to help me envision the entire process.

It is impossible to acknowledge every teacher in my life, but I want to mention some of the most influential physicians who shaped my medical training during my pediatrics residency and allergy/immunology fellowship. They include James Antoon, Andrew Kreppel, Amanda Osta, Michelle Barnes, Lucy Park, Pravin Muniyappa, Brooke Polk, Jeffrey Stokes, Caroline Horner, H. James Wedner, Megan Cooper, Jennifer Monroy, and Leonard Bacharier. Each of these mentors left a lasting impact on how I care for patients, approach clinical challenges, and think critically as both a physician and an educator.

I'm deeply grateful to the exceptional team at Plume for bringing this book to life with such dedication and care. My heartfelt thanks to publisher John Parsley and associate publisher Stephanie Cooper for their guidance and vision; to Jamie Knapp for championing the book as its publicist; to Isabel DaSilva for her thoughtful marketing strategy; and to LeeAnn Pemberton and Dora Mak for shepherding the project through the production process so well. The book's visual appeal owes much to Dominique Jones's striking cover design and Shannon Plunkett's elegant interior layout. I'm also thankful to Patricia Clark for her invaluable legal insight, and to editorial director Jill Schwartzman and assistant editor Charlotte Peters for their expert editorial leadership throughout. Additionally, I'd like to recognize the talented freelancers whose contributions elevated the final product—Paul Girard, for his incredibly informative illustrations, and Joy Simpkins, for her meticulous copyediting.

My family means everything to me. I am so lucky that my immediate family lives nearby and could help me whenever I needed them. My brother and sister-in-law, Jason and Ellen, helped organize playdates and activities with my daughter and their three kids, Samuel, Aden, and Rachel. They helped me get additional free time during the day so that I could finish the book in a timely manner. I'm also incredibly grateful for their constant encouragement, thoughtful advice, and the laughter they've brought into my life throughout this journey.

My grandmother Beverly is in her nineties and is still thriving! I am so lucky that I get to see her every week, and she is the reason why I spent many sleepless nights writing so that I could see her face when she reads these words. Her strength, resilience, and warmth have shaped generations of our family. I love you so much. I wish my grandfather Joseph could have been here to read this book, but I know he is smiling and proud of me from above.

My parents, Ira and Susan, are like no other. They have supported me throughout all my highs and lows in life. Whenever I needed help getting something done, I could call them, and they would be there for me. My dad inspired me to become a doctor, and my mom inspired me to become a compassionate educator. Their unwavering belief in me, even when I doubted myself, has been a constant source of strength. I wouldn't be the person I am today without their love, wisdom, and example.

To my daughter, Juliana, you have inspired me to be the best person I can be. I am incredibly proud of you. I hope all the time I spent writing this book while you were at school, dancing, and swimming classes as well as late nights while you were sleeping help inspire you to achieve your dreams. It could be being a hand doctor, astronaut, lawyer, or anything you put your mind to. If you put in the work, time, and effort, I know you'll accomplish anything! You have a heart full of kindness, a mind full of curiosity, and a spark that lights up every room. All I want is for you to be happy and I love you to the moon and back.

My wife, Melanie, is truly the best person you could ever meet. She has been my rock and has provided me with unwavering support. This book would not have been possible without her. She was the reason that my social media platform was elevated in 2021 and she strongly encouraged me to write this book. Without her love and encouragement, I don't know where I would be. She has sacrificed so much to make sure that I succeed, and I greatly appreciate everything she has done for me. Her strength, patience, and belief in me have carried us through every challenge and triumph. Melanie, I love you with my whole heart and I am excited for our future adventures together.

Bibliography

Chapter 1—The History of Allergies

"Controlled Trial of Effects of Cortisone Acetate in Status Asthmaticus; Report to the Medical Research Council by the Subcommittee on Clinical Trials in Asthma," *The Lancet* 271 (October 1956): 803–6, https://www.ncbi.nlm.nih.gov/pubmed/13368522.

Bahna, S. L., "History of Food Allergy and Where We Are Today," *World Allergy Organization Journal* 17, no. 5 (May 2024), https://doi.org/10.1016/j.waojou.2024.100912.

Bergmann, K.-C., and J. Ring (eds.), *History of Allergy* (Chemical Immunology and Allergy book series, vol. 100) (Karger, 2014).

Bryan, Cyril P., and Heinrich Joachim, *The Papyrus Ebers* (London: Geoffrey Bles, 1930).

Bungy, G. A., J. Mossawi, S. A. Nojoumi et al., "Razi's Report About Seasonal Allergic Rhinitis (Hay Fever) from the 10th Century AD," *International Archives of Allergy and Immunology* 110, no. 3 (1996): 219–24, https://doi.org/10.1159/000237290.

Durham, S. R., and H. Nelson, "Allergen Immunotherapy: A Centenary Celebration," *World Allergy Organization Journal* 4, no. 6 (2011): 104–6, https://doi.org/10.1097/WOX.0b013e3182218920.

Gordon, S., "Elie Metchnikoff, the Man and the Myth," *Journal of Innate Immunology* 8, no. 3 (2016): 223–27, https://doi.org/10.1159/000443331.

Gordon, S., "Phagocytosis: The Legacy of Metchnikoff," *Cell* 166, no. 5 (2016): 1065–68, https://doi.org/10.1016/j.cell.2016.08.017.

Kaufmann, S. H., "Immunology's Foundation: The 100-Year Anniversary of the Nobel Prize to Paul Ehrlich and Elie Metchnikoff," *Nature Immunology* 9, no. 7 (2008): 705–12, https://doi.org/10.1038 /ni0708-705.

Nissim, A., and Y. Chernajovsky, "Historical Development of Monoclonal Antibody Therapeutics," in *Handbook of Experimental Pharmacology*, vol. 181, edited by Y. Chernajovsky and A. Nissim (Springer, 2008): 3–18, https://doi.org/10.1007/978-3-540-73259-4_1.

Page, C., and P. Humphrey, "Sir David Jack: An Extraordinary Drug Discoverer and Developer," *Journal of Clinical Pharmacology* 75, no. 5 (2013): 1213–18, https://doi.org/10.1111/j.1365-2125.2012.04467.x.

Pahor, A. L., and A. Farid, "Ni-Ankh-Sekhmet: First Rhinologist in History," *Journal of Laryngology & Otology* 117, no. 11 (2003): 846–49, https://doi .org/10.1258/002221503322542827.

Platts-Mills, T. A., "The Allergy Epidemics: 1870–2010," *Journal of Allergy and Clinical Immunology* 136, no. 1 (2015): 3–13, https://doi.org/10 .1016/j.jaci.2015.03.048.

Ramachandran, M., and J. K. Aronson, "John Bostock's First Description of Hayfever," *Journal of the Royal Society of Medicine* 104, no. 6 (2011): 237–40, https://doi.org/10.1258/jrsm.2010.10k056.

Rumeau, C., "O Rose Thou Art Sick . . . History of Allergic Rhinitis," *European Annals of Otorhinolaryngology, Head and Neck Diseases* 140, no. 6 (2023): 323–24, https://doi.org/10.1016/j.anorl.2023.10.002.

Sampson, H. A., "Food Allergy: Past, Present and Future," *Allergology International* 65, no. 4 (2016): 363–69, https://doi.org/10.1016/j.alit .2016.08.006.

Smith, M., "Historical and Social Science Perspectives on Food Allergy," *Clinical and Experimental Allergy* 53, no. 9 (2023): 902–10, https://doi .org/10.1111/cea.14360.

Wuthrich, B., "History of Food Allergy," in *History of Allergy*, edited by K.-C. Bergman and J. Ring (Chemical Immunology and Allergy book series, vol. 100) (Karger, 2014): 109–19, https://doi.org/10.1159 /000358616.

Chapter 2—The Immune System

Abbas, A. K., A. H. Lichtman, S. Pillai et al., *Cellular and Molecular Immunology*, 10th ed. (Elsevier, 2021).

Burks, A. W., *Middleton's Allergy: Principles and Practice*, 9th ed. (Elsevier, 2019).

Burton, O. T., J. M. Tamayo, A. J. Stranks et al., "Allergen-Specific IgG Antibody Signaling Through FcγRIIb Promotes Food Tolerance," *Journal of Allergy and Clinical Immunology* 141, no. 1 (2018): 189–201, https://doi.org/10.1016/j.jaci.2017.03.045.

Dudzic, P., D. Chomicz, J. Konczak et al., "Large-Scale Data Mining of Four Billion Human Antibody Variable Regions Reveals Convergence Between Therapeutic and Natural Antibodies That Constrains Search Space for Biologics Drug Discovery," *mAbs* 16, no. 1 (2024): 2361928, https://doi.org/10.1080/19420862.2024.2361928.

Goretzki, A., Y-J. Lin, and S. Schulke, "Immune Metabolism in Allergies, Does It Matter?—A Review of Immune Metabolic Basics and Adaptations Associated with the Activation of Innate Immune Cells in Allergy," *Allergy: European Journal of Allergy and Clinical Immunology* 76, no. 11 (2021): 3314–31, https://doi.org/10.1111/all.14843.

James, L. K., and S. J. Till, "Potential Mechanisms for IgG4 Inhibition of Immediate Hypersensitivity Reactions," *Current Allergy and Asthma Reports* 16, no. 3 (2016): 23, https://doi.org/10.1007/s11882-016-0600-2.

McComb, S., A. Thiriot, B. Akache et al., "Introduction to the Immune System," in *Immunoproteomics*, edited by K. Fulton and S. Twine (Methods in Molecular Biology book series, vol. 2024) (Humana, 2019): 1–24, https://doi.org/10.1007/978-1-4939-9597-4_1.

Nesargikar, P. N., B. Spiller, and R. Chavez, "The Complement System: History, Pathways, Cascade and Inhibitors," *European Journal of Microbiology and Immunology* (Bp) 2, no. 2 (2012): 103–11, https://doi.org/10.1556/EuJMI.2.2012.2.2.

Parkin, J., and B. Cohen, "An Overview of the Immune System," *The Lancet* 357, no. 9270 (2001): 1777–89, https://doi.org/10.1016/S0140-6736(00)04904-7.

Qamar, N., A. B. Fishbein, K. A. Erickson et al., "Naturally Occurring Tolerance Acquisition to Foods in Previously Allergic Children Is Characterized by Antigen Specificity and Associated with Increased Subsets of Regulatory T Cells," *Clinical and Experimental Allergy* 45, no. 11 (2015): 1663–72, https://doi.org/10.1111/cea.12570.

Yatim, K. M., and F. G. Lakkis, "A Brief Journey Through the Immune System," *Clinical Journal of the American Society of Nephrology* 10, no. 7 (2015): 1274–81, https://doi.org/10.2215/CJN.10031014.

Chapter 3—The Anatomy of Allergies

Abbas, A. K., A. H. Lichtman, S. Pillai et al., *Cellular and Molecular Immunology*, 10th ed. (Elsevier, 2021).

Alvord, L. S., and B. L. Farmer, "Anatomy and Orientation of the Human External Ear," *Journal of the American Academy of Audiology* 8, no. 6 (1997): 383–90, https://www.ncbi.nlm.nih.gov/pubmed/9433684.

Bazemore, A. W., and D. R. Smucker, "Lymphadenopathy and Malignancy," *American Family Physician* 66, no. 11 (2002): 2103–10, https://www.ncbi.nlm.nih.gov/pubmed/12484692.

Burks, A. W., *Middleton's Allergy: Principles and Practice*, 9th ed. (Elsevier, 2020).

Bushdid, C., M. O. Magnasco, L. B. Vosshall et al., "Humans Can Discriminate More Than 1 Trillion Olfactory Stimuli," *Science* 343, no. 6177 (2014): 1370–72, https://doi.org/10.1126/science.1249168.

Cole, A. M., P. Dewan, and T. Ganz, "Innate Antimicrobial Activity of Nasal Secretions," *Infection and Immunity* 67, no. 7 (1999): 3267–75, https://doi.org/10.1128/IAI.67.7.3267-3275.1999.

De Troyer, A., and A. M. Boriek, "Mechanics of the Respiratory Muscles," *Comprehensive Physiology* 1, no. 3 (2011): 1273–300, https://doi.org/10.1002/cphy.c100009.

Eby, G. A., "Strong Humming for One Hour Daily to Terminate Chronic Rhinosinusitis in Four Days: A Case Report and Hypothesis for Action by Stimulation of Endogenous Nasal Nitric Oxide Production," *Medical Hypotheses* 66, no. 4 (2006): 851–54, https://doi.org/10.1016/j.mehy.2005.11.035.

Hagbom, M., C. Istrate, D. Engblom et al., "Rotavirus Stimulates Release of Serotonin (5-HT) from Human Enterochromaffin Cells and Activates Brain Structures Involved in Nausea and Vomiting," *PLoS Pathogens* 7, no. 7 (2011): e1002115, https://doi.org/10.1371/journal.ppat.1002115.

Jones, N., "The Nose and Paranasal Sinuses Physiology and Anatomy," *Advances in Drug Delivery Reviews* 51, no. 1–3 (2001): 5–19, https://doi.org/10.1016/s0169-409x(01)00172-7.

Kahana-Zweig, R., M. Geva-Sagiv, A. Weissbrod et al., "Measuring and Characterizing the Human Nasal Cycle," *PLoS One* 11, no. 10 (2016): e0162918, https://doi.org/10.1371/journal.pone.0162918.

Kanitakis, J., "Anatomy, Histology and Immunohistochemistry of Normal Human Skin," *European Journal of Dermatology* 12, no. 4 (2002): 390–99, https://www.ncbi.nlm.nih.gov/pubmed/12095893.

Khan, S., and R. Chang, "Anatomy of the Vestibular System: A Review," *NeuroRehabilitation* 32, no. 3 (2013): 437–43, https://doi.org/10.3233/NRE-130866.

Lorkiewicz-Muszynska, D., W. Kociemba, A. Rewekant et al., "Development of the Maxillary Sinus from Birth to Age 18. Postnatal Growth Pattern," *International Journal of Pediatric Otorhinolaryngology* 79, no. 9 (2015): 1393–400, https://doi.org/10.1016/j.ijporl.2015.05.032.

Marseglia, G. L., D. Poddighe, D. Caimmi et al., "Role of Adenoids and Adenoiditis in Children with Allergy and Otitis Media," *Current Allergy and Asthma Reports* 9, no. 6 (2009): 460–64, https://doi.org/10.1007/s11882-009-0068-4.

McComb, S., A. Thiriot, B. Akache et al., "Introduction to the Immune System," in *Immunoproteomics*, edited by K. Fulton and S. Twine (Methods in Molecular Biology book series, vol. 2024) (Humana, 2019): 1–24, https://doi.org/10.1007/978-1-4939-9597-4_1.

Parkin, J., and B. Cohen, "An Overview of the Immune System," *The Lancet* 357, no. 9270 (2001): 1777–89, https://doi.org/10.1016/S0140-6736(00)04904-7.

Pilarski, J. Q., J. C. Leiter, and R. F. Fregosi, "Muscles of Breathing: Development, Function, and Patterns of Activation," *Comprehensive Physiology* 9, no. 3 (2019): 1025–80, https://doi.org/10.1002/cphy.c180008.

Pynnonen, M. A., M. B. Gillespie, B. Roman et al., "Clinical Practice Guideline: Evaluation of the Neck Mass in Adults," *Otolaryngology—Head and Neck Surgery* 157, no. 2_suppl. (2017): S1–30, https://doi.org/10.1177/0194599817722550.

Quaresma, J. A. S., "Organization of the Skin Immune System and Compartmentalized Immune Responses in Infectious Diseases," *Clinical Microbiology Reviews* 32, no. 4 (2019), https://doi.org/10.1128/CMR.00034-18.

Rubin, B. K., "Physiology of Airway Mucus Clearance," *Respiratory Care* 47, no. 7 (2002): 761–68, https://www.ncbi.nlm.nih.gov/pubmed/12088546.

Voynow, J. A., and B. K. Rubin, "Mucins, Mucus, and Sputum," *Chest* 135, no. 2 (2009): 505–12, https://doi.org/10.1378/chest.08-0412.

Yatim, K. M., and F. G. Lakkis, "A Brief Journey Through the Immune System," *Clinical Journal of the American Society of Nephrology* 10, no. 7 (2015): 1274–81, https://doi.org/10.2215/CJN.10031014.

Zhang, J., Y. Fu, L. Wang et al., "Adenoid Facies: A Long-Term Vicious Cycle of Mouth Breathing, Adenoid Hypertrophy, and Atypical Craniofacial Development," *Frontiers in Public Health* 12 (2024): 1494517, https://doi.org/10.3389/fpubh.2024.1494517.

Chapter 4—What to Expect at the Allergist's Office

Bernstein, I. L., J. T. Li, D. I. Bernstein et al., "Allergy Diagnostic Testing: An Updated Practice Parameter," *Annals of Allergy, Asthma & Immunology* 100, no. 3, Suppl. 3, (2008): S1–148, https://doi.org/10.1016/s1081-1206(10)60305-5.

de Vos, G., "Skin Testing Versus Serum-Specific IgE Testing: Which Is Better for Diagnosing Aeroallergen Sensitization and Predicting Clinical Allergy?" *Current Allergy and Asthma Reports* 14, no. 5 (2014): 430, https://doi.org/10.1007/s11882-014-0430-z.

Dykewicz, M. S., D. V. Wallace, D. J. Amrol et al., "Rhinitis 2020: A Practice Parameter Update," *Journal of Allergy and Clinical Immunology* 146, no. 4 (2020): 721–67, https://doi.org/10.1016/j.jaci.2020.07.007.

Greenhawt, M., M. Shaker, J. Wang et al., "Peanut Allergy Diagnosis: A 2020 Practice Parameter Update, Systematic Review, and GRADE Analysis," *Journal of Allergy and Clinical Immunology* 146, no. 6 (2020): 1302–34, https://doi.org/10.1016/j.jaci.2020.07.031.

Griffiths, R. L. M., T. El-Shanawany, S. R. A. Jolles et al., "Comparison of the Performance of Skin Prick, ImmunoCAP, and ISAC Tests in the Diagnosis of Patients with Allergy," *International Archives of Allergy and Immunology* 172, no. 4 (2017): 215–23, https://doi.org/10.1159/000464326.

Patel, G., and C. Saltoun, "Skin Testing in Allergy," *Allergy & Asthma Proceedings* 40, no. 6 (2019): 366–68, https://doi.org/10.2500/aap.2019.40.4248.

Saah, A. J., and D. R. Hoover, "'Sensitivity' and 'Specificity' Reconsidered: The Meaning of These Terms in Analytical and Diagnostic Settings," *Annals of Internal Medicine* 126, no. 1 (1997): 91–94, https://doi.org/10.7326/0003-4819-126-1-199701010-00026.

Sampson, H. A., S. Aceves, S. A. Bock et al., "Food Allergy: A Practice Parameter Update—2014," *Journal of Allergy and Clinical Immunology* 134, no. 5 (2014): 1016–25.e43, https://doi.org/10.1016/j.jaci.2014.05.013.

Seidman, M. D., R. K. Gurgel, S. Y. Lin et al., "Clinical Practice Guideline: Allergic Rhinitis," *Otolaryngology—Head and Neck Surgery* 152, no. 1 Suppl. (2015): S1–43, https://doi.org/10.1177/0194599814561600.

Soares-Weiser, K., Y. Takwoingi, S. S. Panesar et al., "The Diagnosis of Food Allergy: A Systematic Review and Meta-Analysis," *Allergy: European Journal of Allergy and Clinical Immunology* 69, no. 1 (2014): 76–86, https://doi.org/10.1111/all.12333.

Chapter 5—Allergic Rhinitis and Non-Allergic Rhinitis

United States Department of Agriculture, *Trees: The Yearbook of Agriculture* (US Government Printing Office, 1949).

Akhouri, S., and S. A. House, "Allergic Rhinitis" (StatPearls Publishing), accessed January 1, 2025, https://www.ncbi.nlm.nih.gov/books/NBK538186/.

Bernstein, I. L., J. T. Li, D. I. Bernstein et al., "Allergy Diagnostic Testing: An Updated Practice Parameter," *Annals of Allergy, Asthma & Immunology* 100, no. 3, Suppl. 3 (2008): S1–148, https://doi.org/10.1016/s1081-1206(10)60305-5.

Bjornevik, K., M. Cortese, B. C. Healy et al., "Longitudinal Analysis Reveals High Prevalence of Epstein-Barr Virus Associated with Multiple Sclerosis," *Science* 375, no. 6578 (2022): 296–301, https://doi.org/10.1126/science.abj8222.

Blaiss, M. S., E. O. Meltzer, M. J. Derebery et al., "Patient and Healthcare-Provider Perspectives on the Burden of Allergic Rhinitis," *Allergy Asthma Proceedings* 28, Suppl. 1 (2007): S4–10, https://doi.org/10.2500/aap.2007.28.2991.

Bloomfield, S. F., G. A. Rook, E. A. Scott et al., "Time to Abandon the Hygiene Hypothesis: New Perspectives on Allergic Disease, the Human Microbiome, Infectious Disease Prevention, and the Role of Targeted

Hygiene," *Perspectives in Public Health* 136, no. 4 (2016): 213–24, https://doi.org/10.1177/1757913916650225.

Bloomfield, S. F., R. Stanwell-Smith, R. W. Crevel et al., "Too Clean, or Not Too Clean: The Hygiene Hypothesis and Home Hygiene," *Clinical and Experimental Allergy* 36, no. 4 (2006): 402–25, https://doi.org/10.1111/j.1365-2222.2006.02463.x.

Brawley, A., B. Silverman, S. Kearney et al., "Allergic Rhinitis in Children with Attention-Deficit/Hyperactivity Disorder," *Annals of Allergy, Asthma & Immunology* 92, no. 6 (2004): 663–67, https://doi.org/10.1016/S1081-1206(10)61434-2.

Bremner, S. A., I. M. Carey, S. DeWilde et al., "Infections Presenting for Clinical Care in Early Life and Later Risk of Hay Fever in Two UK Birth Cohorts," *Allergy* 63, no. 3 (2008): 274–83, https://doi.org/10.1111/j.1398-9995.2007.01599.x.

Chapman, M., "Analysis of Dust from the NASA Space Shuttle Revealed Measurable Quantities of Fel D1," paper presented at the Thoracic Society of Australia and New Zealand (TSANZ) meeting (1994).

Dunder, T., T. Tapiainen, T. Pokka et al., "Infections in Child Day Care Centers and Later Development of Asthma, Allergic Rhinitis, and Atopic Dermatitis: Prospective Follow-up Survey 12 Years After Controlled Randomized Hygiene Intervention," *Archives of Pediatrics & Adolescent Medicine* 161, no. 10 (2007): 972–77, https://doi.org/10.1001/archpedi.161.10.972.

Dykewicz, M. S., D. V. Wallace, D. J. Amrol et al., "Rhinitis 2020: A Practice Parameter Update," *Journal of Allergy and Clinical Immunology* 146, no. 4 (2020): 721–67, https://doi.org/10.1016/j.jaci.2020.07.007.

Harris, E., "RSV Infection During Infancy Tied to Asthma Later," *JAMA* 329, no. 20 (2023): 1731, https://doi.org/10.1001/jama.2023.7765.

Jackson, D. J., and J. E. Gern, "Rhinovirus Infections and Their Roles in Asthma: Etiology and Exacerbations," *Journal of Allergy and Clinical Immunology: In Practice* 10, no. 3 (2022): 673–81, https://doi.org/10.1016/j.jaip.2022.01.006.

Kim, K. R., J. W. Oh, S. Y. Woo et al., "Does the Increase in Ambient CO_2 Concentration Elevate Allergy Risks Posed by Oak Pollen?" *International Journal of Biometeorology* 62, no. 9 (2018): 1587–94, https://doi.org/10.1007/s00484-018-1558-7.

Korpela, K., S. Hurley, S. A. Ford et al., "Association Between Gut Microbiota Development and Allergy in Infants Born During Pandemic-Related Social Distancing Restrictions," *Allergy* 79, no. 7 (2024): 1938–51, https://doi.org/10.1111/all.16069.

Lee, Michelle, and Julia Inuma, "Japan's Answer to Seasonal Allergies: A Subsidized Tropical Escape," *Washington Post*, April 4, 2024.

Licari, A., P. Magri, A. De Silvestri et al., "Epidemiology of Allergic Rhinitis in Children: A Systematic Review and Meta-Analysis," *Journal of Allergy and Clinical Immunology: In Practice* 11, no. 8 (2023): 2547–56, https://doi.org/10.1016/j.jaip.2023.05.016.

Marshall, P. S., C. O'Hara, and P. Steinberg, "Effects of Seasonal Allergic Rhinitis on Selected Cognitive Abilities," *Annals of Allergy, Asthma & Immunology* 84, no. 4 (2000): 403–10, https://doi.org/10.1016/S1081-1206(10)62273-9.

Meltzer, E. O., M. S. Blaiss, M. J. Derebery et al., "Burden of Allergic Rhinitis: Results from the Pediatric Allergies in America Survey," *Journal of Allergy and Clinical Immunology* 124, no. 3, Suppl. 1 (2009): S43–70, https://doi.org/10.1016/j.jaci.2009.05.013.

Meltzer, E. O., M. S. Blaiss, R. M. Naclerio et al., "Burden of Allergic Rhinitis: Allergies in America, Latin America, and Asia-Pacific Adult Surveys," *Allergy and Asthma Proceedings* 33, Suppl. 1 (2012): S113–41, https://doi.org/10.2500/aap.2012.33.3603.

Miller, J. D., "The Role of Dust Mites in Allergy," *Clinical Reviews in Allergy & Immunology* 57, no. 3 (2019): 312–29, https://doi.org/10.1007/s12016-018-8693-0.

Nicholas, C. E., G. R. Wegienka, S. L. Havstad et al., "Dog Allergen Levels in Homes with Hypoallergenic Compared with Nonhypoallergenic Dogs," *American Journal of Rhinology & Allergy* 25, no. 4 (2011): 252–56, https://doi.org/10.2500/ajra.2011.25.3606.

Ogren, Thomas, "Botanical Sexism Cultivates Home-Grown Allergies," *Scientific American*, April 29, 2015.

Oh, J., M. Lee, M. Kim et al., "Incident Allergic Diseases in Post-Covid-19 Condition: Multinational Cohort Studies from South Korea, Japan and the UK," *Nature Communications* 15, no. 1 (2024): 2830, https://doi.org/10.1038/s41467-024-47176-w.

Roland, L. T., S. K. Wise, H. Wang et al., "The Cost of Rhinitis in the United States: A National Insurance Claims Analysis," *International Forum of*

Allergy & Rhinology 11, no. 5 (2021): 946–48, https://doi
.org/10.1002/alr.22748.

Satyaraj, E., C. Gardner, I. Filipi et al., "Reduction of Active Fel D1 from
Cats Using an AntiFel D1 Egg IgY Antibody," *Immunology and
Inflammation Diseases* 7, no. 2 (2019): 68–73, https://doi.org/10.1002
/iid3.244.

Satyaraj, E., H. J. Wedner, and J. Bousquet, "Keep the Cat, Change the Care
Pathway: A Transformational Approach to Managing Fel D 1, the Major
Cat Allergen," *Allergy* 74, Suppl. 107 (2019): 5–17, https://doi
.org/10.1111/all.14013.

Thavagnanam, S., J. Fleming, A. Bromley et al., "A Meta-Analysis of the
Association Between Caesarean Section and Childhood Asthma," *Clinical
and Experimental Allergy* 38, no. 4 (2008): 629–33, https://doi.org
/10.1111/j.1365-2222.2007.02780.x.

Vandenplas, O., D. Vinnikov, P. D. Blanc et al., "Impact of Rhinitis on Work
Productivity: A Systematic Review," *Journal of Allergy and Clinical
Immunology: In Practice* 6, no. 4 (2018): 1274–86 e9, https://doi.org
/10.1016/j.jaip.2017.09.002.

Wood, R. A., M. D. Chapman, N. F. Adkinson Jr. et al., "The Effect of Cat
Removal on Allergen Content in Household-Dust Samples," *Journal of
Allergy and Clinical Immunology* 83, no. 4 (1989): 730–34, https://doi
.org/10.1016/0091-6749(89)90006-7.

Zhang, Y., and A. L. Steiner, "Projected Climate-Driven Changes in Pollen
Emission Season Length and Magnitude over the Continental United
States," *Nature Communications* 13, no. 1 (2022): 1234, https://doi.org
/10.1038/s41467-022-28764-0.

Ziska, L. H., L. Makra, S. K. Harry et al., "Temperature-Related
Changes in Airborne Allergenic Pollen Abundance and Seasonality Across
the Northern Hemisphere: A Retrospective Data Analysis," *Lancet
Planetary Health* 3, no. 3 (2019): e124–31, https://doi.org/10.1016
/S2542-5196(19)30015-4.

Chapter 6—Sinusitis

Berges-Gimeno, M. P., R. A. Simon, and D. D. Stevenson, "Long-Term
Treatment with Aspirin Desensitization in Asthmatic Patients with
Aspirin-Exacerbated Respiratory Disease," *Journal of Allergy and
Clinical Immunology* 111, no. 1 (2003): 180–86, https://doi.org/10
.1067/mai.2003.7.

Blackwell, D. L., J. W. Lucas, and T. C. Clarke, "Summary Health Statistics for U.S. Adults: National Health Interview Survey, 2012," *Vital and Health Statistics* 10 (2014): 1–161, https://www.ncbi.nlm.nih.gov/pubmed/24819891.

Calvo-Henriquez, C., E. Di Corso, I. Alobid et al., "Pathophysiological Link Between Chronic Rhinosinusitis and Ear Disease," *Current Allergy and Asthma Reports* 23, no. 7 (2023): 389–97, https://doi.org/10.1007/s11882-023-01072-3.

Cardet, J. C., A. A. White, N. A. Barrett et al., "Alcohol-Induced Respiratory Symptoms Are Common in Patients with Aspirin Exacerbated Respiratory Disease," *Journal of Allergy and Clinical Immunology: In Practice* 2, no. 2 (2014): 208–13, https://doi.org/10.1016/j.jaip.2013.12.003.

DeMuri, G. P., J. C. Eickhoff, J. C. Gern et al., "Clinical and Virological Characteristics of Acute Sinusitis in Children," *Clinical Infectious Diseases* 69, no. 10 (2019): 1764–70, https://doi.org/10.1093/cid/ciz023.

DeMuri, G. P., J. E. Gern, S. C. Moyer et al., "Clinical Features, Virus Identification, and Sinusitis as a Complication of Upper Respiratory Tract Illness in Children Ages 4–7 Years," *Journal of Pediatrics* 171 (2016): 133–39 e1, https://doi.org/10.1016/j.jpeds.2015.12.034.

Fahrenholz, J. M., "Natural History and Clinical Features of Aspirin-Exacerbated Respiratory Disease," *Clinical Reviews in Allergy & Immunology* 24, no. 2 (2003): 113–24, https://doi.org/10.1385/CRIAI:24:2:113.

Fokkens, W. J., V. J. Lund, C. Hopkins et al., "European Position Paper on Rhinosinusitis and Nasal Polyps 2020," *Rhinology* 58, Suppl. 29 (2020): S1–464, https://doi.org/10.4193/Rhin20.600.

Hope, A. P., K. A. Woessner, R. A. Simon et al., "Rational Approach to Aspirin Dosing During Oral Challenges and Desensitization of Patients with Aspirin-Exacerbated Respiratory Disease," *Journal of Allergy and Clinical Immunology* 123, no. 2 (2009): 406–10, https://doi.org/10.1016/j.jaci.2008.09.048.

Huang, D., M. S. Taha, A. L. Nocera et al., "Cold Exposure Impairs Extracellular Vesicle Swarm-Mediated Nasal Antiviral Immunity," *Journal of Allergy and Clinical Immunology* 151, no. 2 (2023): 509–25 e8, https://doi.org/10.1016/j.jaci.2022.09.037.

Jani, A. L., and D. L. Hamilos, "Current Thinking on the Relationship Between Rhinosinusitis and Asthma," *Journal of Asthma* 42, no. 1 (2005): 1–7, https://doi.org/10.1081/jas-200044744.

Kim, Y. S., N. H. Kim, S. Y. Seong et al., "Prevalence and Risk Factors of Chronic Rhinosinusitis in Korea," *American Journal of Rhinology & Allergy* 25, no. 3 (2011): 117–21, https://doi.org/10.2500/ajra.2011.25.3630.

Klossek, J. M., F. Neukirch, C. Pribil et al., "Prevalence of Nasal Polyposis in France: A Cross-Sectional, Case-Control Study," *Allergy: European Journal of Allergy and Clinical Immunology* 60, no. 2 (2005): 233–37, https://doi.org/10.1111/j.1398-9995.2005.00688.x.

Kowalski, M. L., R. Pawliczak, J. Wozniak et al., "Differential Metabolism of Arachidonic Acid in Nasal Polyp Epithelial Cells Cultured from Aspirin-Sensitive and Aspirin-Tolerant Patients," *American Journal of Respiratory and Critical Care Medicine* 161, no. 2, Pt. 1 (2000): 391–98, https://doi.org/10.1164/ajrccm.161.2.9902034.

Lambrakis, P., G. F. Rushworth, J. Adamson et al., "Aspirin Hypersensitivity and Desensitization Protocols: Implications for Cardiac Patients," *Therapeutic Advances in Drug Safety* 2, no. 6 (2011): 263–70, https://doi.org/10.1177/2042098611422558.

Lang, D. M., M. A. Aronica, E. S. Maierson et al., "Omalizumab Can Inhibit Respiratory Reaction During Aspirin Desensitization," *Annals of Allergy, Asthma & Immunology* 121, no. 1 (2018): 98–104, https://doi.org/10.1016/j.anai.2018.05.007.

Marom, T., P. E. Alvarez-Fernandez, K. Jennings et al., "Acute Bacterial Sinusitis Complicating Viral Upper Respiratory Tract Infection in Young Children," *Pediatric Infectious Disease Journal* 33, no. 8 (2014): 803–8, https://doi.org/10.1097/INF.0000000000000278.

Mustafa, S. S., and K. Vadamalai, "Dupilumab Increases Aspirin Tolerance in Aspirin-Exacerbated Respiratory Disease," *Annals of Allergy, Asthma & Immunology* 126, no. 6 (2021): 738–39, https://doi.org/10.1016/j.anai.2021.03.010.

Payne, S. C., and M. S. Benninger, "Staphylococcus Aureus Is a Major Pathogen in Acute Bacterial Rhinosinusitis: A Meta-Analysis," *Clinical Infectious Diseases* 45, no. 10 (2007): e121–27, https://doi.org/10.1086/522763.

Peters, A. T., S. Spector, J. Hsu et al., "Diagnosis and Management of Rhinosinusitis: A Practice Parameter Update," *Annals of Allergy, Asthma*

& *Immunology* 113, no. 4 (2014): 347–85, https://doi.org
/10.1016/j.anai.2014.07.025.

Rajan, J. P., N. E. Wineinger, D. D. Stevenson et al., "Prevalence of Aspirin-
Exacerbated Respiratory Disease Among Asthmatic Patients: A Meta-
Analysis of the Literature," *Journal of Allergy and Clinical Immunology*
135, no. 3 (2015): 676–81 e1, https://doi.org/10.1016/j.jaci
.2014.08.020.

Rank, M. A., D. K. Chu, A. Bognanni et al., "The Joint Task Force on Practice
Parameters Grade Guidelines for the Medical Management of Chronic
Rhinosinusitis with Nasal Polyposis," *Journal of Allergy and Clinical
Immunology* 151, no. 2 (2023): 386–98, https://doi.org/10.1016
/j.jaci.2022.10.026.

Rosenfeld, R. M., J. F. Piccirillo, S. S. Chandrasekhar, et al., "Clinical
Practice Guideline (Update): Adult Sinusitis," *Otolaryngology—Head
and Neck Surgery* 152, no. 2 Suppl. (2015): S1–39, https://doi.org/10
.1177/0194599815572097.

Schlosser, R. J., S. E. Gage, P. Kohli et al., "Burden of Illness: A Systematic
Review of Depression in Chronic Rhinosinusitis," *American Journal of
Rhinology & Allergy* 30, no. 4 (2016): 250–56, https://doi.org/10.2500
/ajra.2016.30.4343.

Smith, T. L., R. J. Schlosser, J. C. Mace et al., "Long-Term Outcomes of
Endoscopic Sinus Surgery in the Management of Adult Chronic
Rhinosinusitis," *International Forum of Allergy & Rhinology* 9, no. 8
(2019): 831–41, https://doi.org/10.1002/alr.22369.

Venekamp, R. P., M. J. Thompson, G. Hayward et al., "Systemic
Corticosteroids for Acute Sinusitis," *Cochrane Database of Systematic
Reviews,* no. 3 (2014): CD008115, https://doi.org/10.1002/14651858
.CD008115.pub3.

Chapter 7—Food Allergies

American Academy of Pediatrics, Committee on Nutrition, "Hypoallergenic
Infant Formulas," *Pediatrics* 106, no. 2, Pt. 1 (2000): 346–49, https://
www.ncbi.nlm.nih.gov/pubmed/10920165.

Codex Alimentarius Commission (CAC), "Work of the Codex Committee on
Food Labelling," 47th Session of the CAC, 2024, https://www.fao
.org/fao-who-codexalimentarius/meetings/detail/en/?meeting=CAC&
session=47.

Allen, K. J., J. J. Koplin, A. L. Ponsonby et al., "Vitamin D Insufficiency Is Associated with Challenge-Proven Food Allergy in Infants," *Journal of Allergy and Clinical Immunology* 131, no. 4 (2013): 1109–16, 16 e1–6, https://doi.org/10.1016/j.jaci.2013.01.017.

Azad, M. B., T. Konya, D. S. Guttman et al., "Infant Gut Microbiota and Food Sensitization: Associations in the First Year of Life," *Clinical and Experimental Allergy* 45, no. 3 (2015): 632–43, https://doi.org/10.1111/cea.12487.

Cooke, F., A. Ramos, and L. Herbert, "Food Allergy-Related Bullying Among Children and Adolescents," *Journal of Pediatric Psychology* 47, no. 3 (2022): 318–26, https://doi.org/10.1093/jpepsy/jsab099.

Du Toit, G., G. Roberts, P. H. Sayre et al., "Randomized Trial of Peanut Consumption in Infants at Risk for Peanut Allergy," *New England Journal of Medicine* 372, no. 9 (2015): 803–13, https://doi.org/10.1056/NEJMoa1414850.

Du Toit, G., M. F. Huffaker, S. Radulovic et al., "Follow-up to Adolescence After Early Peanut Introduction for Allergy Prevention," *New England Journal of Medicine: Evidence* 3, no. 6 (2024): EVIDoa2300311, https://doi.org/10.1056/EVIDoa2300311.

Ginde, A. A., M. C. Liu, and C. A. Camargo Jr., "Demographic Differences and Trends of Vitamin D Insufficiency in the US Population, 1988–2004," *Archives of Internal Medicine* 169, no. 6 (2009): 626–32, https://doi.org/10.1001/archinternmed.2008.604.

Greer, F. R., S. H. Sicherer, A. W. Burks et al., "The Effects of Early Nutritional Interventions on the Development of Atopic Disease in Infants and Children: The Role of Maternal Dietary Restriction, Breastfeeding, Hydrolyzed Formulas, and Timing of Introduction of Allergenic Complementary Foods," *Pediatrics* 143, no. 4 (2019), https://doi.org/10.1542/peds.2019-0281.

Gupta, R. S., C. M. Warren, B. M. Smith et al., "The Public Health Impact of Parent-Reported Childhood Food Allergies in the United States," *Pediatrics* 142, no. 6 (2018), https://doi.org/10.1542/peds.2018-1235.

Gupta, R. S., C. M. Warren, B. M. Smith et al., "Prevalence and Severity of Food Allergies Among US Adults," *JAMA Network Open* 2, no. 1 (2019): e185630, https:// doi.org/ 10.1001/ jamanetworkopen.2018.5630.

Hirano, I., E. S. Chan, M. A. Rank et al., "AGA Institute and the Joint Task Force on Allergy-Immunology Practice Parameters Clinical Guidelines for the Management of Eosinophilic Esophagitis," *Annals of Allergy, Asthma & Immunology* 124, no. 5 (2020): 416–23, https://doi.org/10.1016/j.anai.2020.03.020.

Hourihane, J. O., K. J. Allen, W. G. Shreffler et al., "Peanut Allergen Threshold Study (PATS): Novel Single-Dose Oral Food Challenge Study to Validate Eliciting Doses in Children with Peanut Allergy," *Journal of Allergy and Clinical Immunology* 139, no. 5 (2017): 1583–90, https://doi.org/10.1016/j.jaci.2017.01.030.

Iweala, O. I., S. K. Choudhary, and S. P. Commins, "Food Allergy," *Current Gastroenterology Reports* 20, no. 5 (2018): 17, https://doi.org/10.1007/s11894-018-0624-y.

Jackson, K. D., L. D. Howie, and L. J. Akinbami, "Trends in Allergic Conditions Among Children: United States, 1997–2011," NCHS Data Brief no. 121 (2013): 1–8, https://www.ncbi.nlm.nih.gov/pubmed/23742874.

Kato, Y., T. Morikawa, and S. Fujieda, "Comprehensive Review of Pollen-Food Allergy Syndrome: Pathogenesis, Epidemiology, and Treatment Approaches," *Allergology International* 74, no. 1 (2025): 42–50, https://doi.org/10.1016/j.alit.2024.08.007.

Lavine, E., "Blood Testing for Sensitivity, Allergy or Intolerance to Food," *Canadian Medical Association Journal* 184, no. 6 (2012): 666–68, https://doi.org/10.1503/cmaj.110026.

Lee, E., D. E. Campbell, E. H. Barnes et al., "Resolution of Acute Food Protein-Induced Enterocolitis Syndrome in Children," *Journal of Allergy and Clinical Immunology: In Practice* 5, no. 2 (2017): 486–88, e1, https://doi.org/10.1016/j.jaip.2016.09.032.

Martin, P. E., J. K. Eckert, J. J. Koplin et al., "Which Infants with Eczema Are at Risk of Food Allergy? Results from a Population-Based Cohort," *Clinical and Experimental Allergy* 45, no. 1 (2015): 255–64, https://doi.org/10.1111/cea.12406.

Parrish, C. P., "A Review of Food Allergy Panels and Their Consequences," *Annals of Allergy, Asthma & Immunology* 131, no. 4 (2023): 421–26, https://doi.org/10.1016/j.anai.2023.04.011.

Patel, R., and A. P. Koterba, "Peanut Allergy" (StatPearls Publishing, 2023), accessed January 1, 2025, https://www.ncbi.nlm.nih.gov/books/NBK538526/.

Radke, T. J., L. G. Brown, B. Faw et al., "Restaurant Food Allergy Practices—Six Selected Sites, United States, 2014," *MMWR Morbidity and Mortality Weekly Report* 66, no. 15 (2017): 404–7, https://doi.org/10.15585/mmwr.mm6615a2.

Redd, W. D., and E. S. Dellon, "Eosinophilic Gastrointestinal Diseases Beyond the Esophagus: An Evolving Field and Nomenclature," *Gastroenterology & Hepatology* 18, no. 9 (2022): 522–28, https://www.ncbi.nlm.nih.gov/pubmed/36397988.

Shah, S., R. Grohman, and A. Nowak-Wegrzyn, "Food Protein-Induced Enterocolitis Syndrome (FPIES): Beyond the Guidelines," *Journal of Food Allergy* 5, no. 2 (2023): 55–64, https://doi.org/10.2500/jfa.2023.5.230014.

Sharief, S., S. Jariwala, J. Kumar et al., "Vitamin D Levels and Food and Environmental Allergies in the United States: Results from the National Health and Nutrition Examination Survey 2005–2006," *Journal of Allergy and Clinical Immunology* 127, no. 5 (2011): 1195–202, https://doi.org/10.1016/j.jaci.2011.01.017.

Sicherer, S. H., A. W. Burks, and H. A. Sampson, "Clinical Features of Acute Allergic Reactions to Peanut and Tree Nuts in Children," *Pediatrics* 102, no. 1 (1998): e6, https://doi.org/10.1542/peds.102.1.e6.

Singh, A. B., and P. Kumar, "Climate Change and Allergic Diseases: An Overview," *Frontiers in Allergy* 3 (2022): 964987, https://doi.org/10.3389/falgy.2022.964987.

Smith, P. K., J. O. Hourihane, and P. Lieberman, "Risk Multipliers for Severe Food Anaphylaxis," *World Allergy Organization Journal* 8, no. 1 (2015): 30, https://doi.org/10.1186/s40413-015-0081-0.

Thivalapill, N., A. B. Andy-Nweye, L. A. Bilaver et al., "Sensitization to House Dust Mite and Cockroach May Mediate the Racial Difference in Shellfish Allergy," *Pediatric Allergy and Immunology* 33, no. 8 (2022): e13837, https://doi.org/10.1111/pai.13837.

Zablotsky, B., L. I. Black, and L. J. Akinbami, "Diagnosed Allergic Conditions in Children Aged 0–17 Years: United States, 2021," *NCHS Data Brief* no. 459 (2023): 1–8, https://www.ncbi.nlm.nih.gov/pubmed/36700870.

Chapter 8—Eczema

AAAAI/ACAAI JTF Atopic Dermatitis Guideline Panel, D. K. Chu, L. Schneider, R. N. Asiniwasis et al., "Atopic Dermatitis (Eczema) Guidelines: 2023 American Academy of Allergy, Asthma and

Immunology/American College of Allergy, Asthma and Immunology Joint Task Force on Practice Parameters Grade– and Institute of Medicine–Based Recommendations," *Annals of Allergy, Asthma & Immunology* 132, no. 3 (2024): 274–312, https://doi.org/10.1016 /j.anai.2023.11.009.

Abuabara, K., D. J. Margolis, and S. M. Langan, "The Long-Term Course of Atopic Dermatitis," *Dermatologic Clinics* 35, no. 3 (2017): 291–97, https://doi.org/10.1016/j.det.2017.02.003.

Chen, Y. T., and H. Y. Chiu, "Short-Term Risks of Major Adverse Cardiovascular Events Associated with Janus Kinase Inhibitors in Patients with Atopic Dermatitis: A Systematic Review and Meta-Analysis," *Journal of the European Academy of Dermatology and Venereology* 37, no. 8: e1055–58, https://doi.org/10.1111/jdv.19102.

Chiesa Fuxench, Z. C., J. K. Block, M. Boguniewicz et al., "Atopic Dermatitis in America Study: A Cross-Sectional Study Examining the Prevalence and Disease Burden of Atopic Dermatitis in the US Adult Population," *Journal of Investigative Dermatology* 139, no. 3 (2019): 583–90, https://doi.org /10.1016/j.jid.2018.08.028.

Chiesa Fuxench, Z. C., N. Mitra, D. Del Pozo et al., "Risk of Atopic Dermatitis and the Atopic March Paradigm in Children of Mothers with Atopic Illnesses: A Birth Cohort Study from the United Kingdom," *Journal of the American Academy of Dermatology* 90, no. 3 (2024): 561–68, https://doi .org/10.1016/j.jaad.2023.11.013.

Czarnowicki, T., H. He, J. G. Krueger et al., "Atopic Dermatitis Endotypes and Implications for Targeted Therapeutics," *Journal of Allergy and Clinical Immunology* 143, no. 1 (2019): 1–11, https://doi.org/10.1016/j .jaci.2018.10.032.

Dahlsgaard, K. K., M. O. Lewis, and J. M. Spergel, "New Issue of Food Allergy: Phobia of Anaphylaxis in Pediatric Patients," *Journal of Allergy and Clinical Immunology* 146, no. 4 (2020): 780–82, https://doi.org/10.1016 /j.jaci.2020.07.010.

Datsi, A., M. Steinhoff, F. Ahmad et al., "Interleukin-31: The 'Itchy' Cytokine in Inflammation and Therapy," *Allergy: European Journal of Allergy and Clinical Immunology* 76, no. 10 (2021): 2982–97, https://doi.org/10.1111 /all.14791.

David, T. J., and M. Longson, "Herpes Simplex Infections in Atopic Eczema," *Archives of Disease in Childhood* 60, no. 4 (1985): 338–43, https://doi.org /10.1136/adc.60.4.338.

Deckers, I. A., S. McLean, S. Linssen et al., "Investigating International Time Trends in the Incidence and Prevalence of Atopic Eczema 1990–2010: A Systematic Review of Epidemiological Studies," *PLoS One* 7, no. 7 (2012): e39803, https://doi.org/10.1371/journal.pone.0039803.

Deng, L., F. Costa, K. J. Blake et al., "*S. Aureus* Drives Itch and Scratch-Induced Skin Damage Through a V8 Protease-Par1 Axis," *Cell* 186, no. 24 (2023): 5375–93 e25, https://doi.org/10.1016/j.cell.2023.10.019.

Geoghegan, J. A., A. D. Irvine, and T. J. Foster, "*Staphylococcus Aureus* and Atopic Dermatitis: A Complex and Evolving Relationship," *Trends in Microbiology* 26, no. 6 (2018): 484–97, https://doi.org/10.1016/j.tim.2017.11.008.

Ingrassia, J. P., M. H. Maqsood, J. M. Gelfand et al., "Cardiovascular and Venous Thromboembolic Risk with Jak Inhibitors in Immune-Mediated Inflammatory Skin Diseases: A Systematic Review and Meta-Analysis," *JAMA Dermatology* 160, no. 1 (2024): 28–36, https://doi.org/10.1001/jamadermatol.2023.4090.

Katibi, O. S., M. J. Cork, C. Flohr et al., "Moisturizer Therapy in Prevention of Atopic Dermatitis and Food Allergy: To Use or Disuse?" *Annals of Allergy, Asthma & Immunology* 128, no. 5 (2022): 512–25, https://doi.org/10.1016/j.anai.2022.02.012.

Keet, C., M. Pistiner, M. Plesa et al., "Age and Eczema Severity, but Not Family History, Are Major Risk Factors for Peanut Allergy in Infancy," *Journal of Allergy and Clinical Immunology* 147, no. 3 (2021): 984–91 e5, https://doi.org/10.1016/j.jaci.2020.11.033.

Kim, J. P., L. X. Chao, E. L. Simpson et al., "Persistence of Atopic Dermatitis (AD): A Systematic Review and Meta-Analysis," *Journal of the American Academy of Dermatology* 75, no. 4 (2016): 681–87 e11, https://doi.org/10.1016/j.jaad.2016.05.028.

Luschkova, D., K. Zeiser, A. Ludwig et al., "Atopic Eczema Is an Environmental Disease," *Allergology Select* 5, no. 1 (2021): 244–50, https://doi.org/10.5414/ALX02258E.

Mohn, C. H., H. S. Blix, J. A. Halvorsen et al., "Incidence Trends of Atopic Dermatitis in Infancy and Early Childhood in a Nationwide Prescription Registry Study in Norway," *JAMA Network Open* 1, no. 7 (2018): e184145, https://doi.org/10.1001/jamanetworkopen.2018.4145.

Odhiambo, J. A., H. C. Williams, T. O. Clayton et al., "Global Variations in Prevalence of Eczema Symptoms in Children from Isaac Phase Three,"

Journal of Allergy and Clinical Immunology 124, no. 6 (2009): 1251–58 e23, https://doi.org/10.1016/j.jaci.2009.10.009.

Oykhman, P., J. Dookie, H. Al-Rammahy et al., "Dietary Elimination for the Treatment of Atopic Dermatitis: A Systematic Review and Meta-Analysis," *Journal of Allergy and Clinical Immunology: In Practice* 10, no. 10 (2022): 2657–66 e8, https://doi.org/10.1016/j.jaip.2022.06.044.

Rendell, M. E., S. F. Baig-Lewis, T. M. Berry et al., "Do Early Skin Care Practices Alter the Risk of Atopic Dermatitis? A Case-Control Study," *Pediatric Dermatology* 28, no. 5 (2011): 593–95, https://doi.org/10.1111/j.1525-1470.2011.01384.x.

Schafer, T., J. Heinrich, M. Wjst et al., "Association Between Severity of Atopic Eczema and Degree of Sensitization to Aeroallergens in Schoolchildren," *Journal of Allergy and Clinical Immunology* 104, no. 6 (1999): 1280–84, https://doi.org/10.1016/s0091-6749(99)70025-4.

Silverberg, J. I., S. Barbarot, A. Gadkari et al., "Atopic Dermatitis in the Pediatric Population: A Cross-Sectional, International Epidemiologic Study," *Annals of Allergy, Asthma & Immunology* 126, no. 4 (2021): 417–28 e2, https://doi.org/10.1016/j.anai.2020.12.020.

Weare-Regales, N., S. E. Chiarella, J. C. Cardet et al., "Hormonal Effects on Asthma, Rhinitis, and Eczema," *Journal of Allergy and Clinical Immunology in Practice* 10, no. 8 (2022): 2066–73, https://doi.org/10.1016/j.jaip.2022.04.002.

Wheeler, C. E., Jr., and D. C. Abele, "Eczema Herpeticum, Primary and Recurrent," *Archives of Dermatology* 93, no. 2 (1966): 162–73, https://doi.org/10.1001/archderm.1966.01600200018002.

Ytterberg, S. R., D. L. Bhatt, T. R. Mikuls et al., "Cardiovascular and Cancer Risk with Tofacitinib in Rheumatoid Arthritis," *New England Journal of Medicine* 386, no. 4 (2022): 313–26, https://doi.org/10.1056/NEJMoa 2109927.

Chapter 9—Contact Dermatitis

Ahlstrom, M. G., J. P. Thyssen, T. Menne et al., "Prevalence of Nickel Allergy in Europe Following the EU Nickel Directive—A Review," *Contact Dermatitis* 77, no. 4 (2017): 193–200, https://doi.org/10.1111/cod.12846.

Aquino, M. R., K. Schmidlin, and C. M. Woodruff, "Managing Contact Dermatitis Without Patch Testing," *Journal of Allergy and Clinical*

Immunology: In Practice 12, no. 9 (2024): 2252–59, https://doi.org/10 .1016/j.jaip.2024.04.047.

Beltrani, V. S., and V. P. Beltrani, "Contact Dermatitis," *Annals of Allergy, Asthma & Immunology* 78, no. 2 (1997): 160–73, quiz 174–76, https://doi.org/10.1016/S1081-1206(10)63383-2.

Crane, M. M., D. J. Webb, E. Watson et al., "Hand Eczema and Steroid-Refractory Chronic Hand Eczema in General Practice: Prevalence and Initial Treatment," *British Journal of Dermatology* 176, no. 4 (2017): 955–64, https://doi.org/10.1111/bjd.14974.

Cunningham, E., "What Role Does Diet Play in the Management of Nickel Allergy?" *Journal of the Academy of Nutrition and Dietetics* 117, no. 3 (2017): 500, https://doi.org/10.1016/j.jand.2017.01.001.

Diepgen, T. L., R. F. Ofenloch, M. Bruze et al., "Prevalence of Contact Allergy in the General Population in Different European Regions," *British Journal of Dermatology* 174, no. 2 (2016): 319–29, https://doi .org/10.1111/bjd.14167.

Fabbro, S. K., and M. J. Zirwas, "Systemic Contact Dermatitis to Foods: Nickel, BOP, and More," *Current Allergy and Asthma Reports* 14, no. 10 (2014): 463, https://doi.org/10.1007/s11882-014 -0463-3.

Fonacier, L., D. I. Bernstein, K. Pacheco et al., "Contact Dermatitis: A Practice Parameter—Update 2015," *Journal of Allergy and Clinical Immunology: In Practice* 3, no. 3 Suppl. (2015): S1–39, https://doi.org /10.1016/j.jaip.2015.02.009.

Fowler, J. F., Jr., "Cobalt," *Dermatitis* 27, no. 1 (2016): 3–8, https://doi.org /10.1097/DER.0000000000000154.

Fransway, A. F., P. J. Fransway, D. V. Belsito et al., "Paraben Toxicology," *Dermatitis* 30, no. 1 (2019): 32–45, https://doi.org/10.1097/DER .0000000000000428.

Genchi, G., G. Lauria, A. Catalano et al., "Prevalence of Cobalt in the Environment and Its Role in Biological Processes," *Biology* 12, no. 10 (2023): 1335, https://doi.org/10.3390/biology12101335.

Hiranput, S., L. McAllister, G. Hill et al., "Do Hypoallergenic Skincare Products Contain Fewer Potential Contact Allergens?" *Clinical and Experimental Dermatology* 49, no. 4 (2024): 386–87, https://doi.org/10 .1093/ced/llad436.

Malkonen, T., K. Alanko, R. Jolanki et al., "Long-Term Follow-up Study of Occupational Hand Eczema," *British Journal of Dermatology* 163, no. 5 (2010): 999–1006, https://doi.org/10.1111/j.1365-2133.2010.09987.x.

McFadden, J., "Immunologic Contact Urticaria," *Immunology and Allergy Clinics of North America* 34, no. 1 (2014): 157–67, https://doi.org/10.1016/j.iac.2013.09.005.

Militello, M., S. Hu, M. Laughter et al., "American Contact Dermatitis Society Allergens of the Year 2000 to 2020," *Dermatologic Clinics* 38, no. 3 (2020): 309–20, https://doi.org/10.1016/j.det.2020.02.011.

Mortz, C. G., and K. E. Andersen, "Allergic Contact Dermatitis in Children and Adolescents," *Contact Dermatitis* 41, no. 3 (1999): 121–30, https://doi.org/10.1111/j.1600-0536.1999.tb06102.x.

Rolls, S., S. Rajan, A. Shah et al., "(Meth)Acrylate Allergy: Frequently Missed?" *British Journal of Dermatology* 178, no. 4 (2018): 980–81, https://doi.org/10.1111/bjd.16402.

Scheman, A., S. Hylwa-Deufel, S. E. Jacob et al., "Alternatives for Allergens in the 2018 American Contact Dermatitis Society Core Series: Report by the American Contact Alternatives Group," *Dermatitis* 30, no. 2 (2019): 87–105, https://doi.org/10.1097/DER.0000000000000453.

Suneja, T., K. H. Flanagan, and D. A. Glaser, "Blue-Jean Button Nickel: Prevalence and Prevention of Its Release from Buttons," *Dermatitis* 18, no. 4 (2007): 208–11, https://doi.org/10.2310/6620.2007.07013.

Thyssen, J. P., J. D. Johansen, A. Linneberg et al., "The Epidemiology of Hand Eczema in the General Population—Prevalence and Main Findings," *Contact Dermatitis* 62, no. 2 (2010): 75–87, https://doi.org/10.1111/j.1600-0536.2009.01669.x.

Usatine, R. P., and M. Riojas, "Diagnosis and Management of Contact Dermatitis," *American Family Physician* 82, no. 3 (2010): 249–55, https://www.ncbi.nlm.nih.gov/pubmed/20672788.

Warshaw, E. M., N. C. Botto, K. A. Zug et al., "Contact Dermatitis Associated with Food: Retrospective Cross-Sectional Analysis of North American Contact Dermatitis Group Data, 2001–2004," *Dermatitis* 19, no. 5 (2008): 252–60, https://www.ncbi.nlm.nih.gov/pubmed/18845115.

Yoshihisa, Y., and T. Shimizu, "Metal Allergy and Systemic Contact Dermatitis: An Overview," *Dermatology Research and Practice* 2012 (2012): 749561, https://doi.org/10.1155/2012/749561.

Chapter 10—Urticaria and Angioedema

Agostoni, A., E. Aygoren-Pursun, K. E. Binkley et al., "Hereditary and Acquired Angioedema: Problems and Progress: Proceedings of the Third C1 Esterase Inhibitor Deficiency Workshop and Beyond," *Journal of Allergy and Clinical Immunology* 114, no. 3 Suppl. (2004): S51–131, https://doi.org/10.1016/j.jaci.2004.06.047.

Alangari, A. A., F. J. Twarog, M. C. Shih et al., "Clinical Features and Anaphylaxis in Children with Cold Urticaria," *Pediatrics* 113, no. 4 (2004): e313–17, https://doi.org/10.1542/peds.113.4.e313.

Barniol, C., E. Dehours, J. Mallet et al., "Levocetirizine and Prednisone Are Not Superior to Levocetirizine Alone for the Treatment of Acute Urticaria: A Randomized Double-Blind Clinical Trial," *Annals of Emergency Medicine* 71, no. 1 (2018): 125–31 e1, https://doi.org/10.1016/j.annemergmed.2017.03.006.

Bernstein, J. A., D. M. Lang, D. A. Khan et al., "The Diagnosis and Management of Acute and Chronic Urticaria: 2014 Update," *Journal of Allergy and Clinical Immunology* 133, no. 5 (2014): 1270–77, https://doi.org/10.1016/j.jaci.2014.02.036.

Bizjak, M., M. Kosnik, D. Dinevski et al., "Risk Factors for Systemic Reactions in Typical Cold Urticaria: Results from the COLD-CE Study," *Allergy: European Journal of Allergy and Clinical Immunology* 77, no. 7 (2022): 2185–99, https://doi.org/10.1111/all.15194.

Bork, K., "Diagnosis and Treatment of Hereditary Angioedema with Normal C1 Inhibitor," *Allergy, Asthma & Clinical Immunology* 6, no. 1 (2010): 15, https://doi.org/10.1186/1710-1492-6-15.

Frank, M. M., J. A. Gelfand, and J. P. Atkinson, "Hereditary Angioedema: The Clinical Syndrome and Its Management," *Annals of Internal Medicine* 84, no. 5 (1976): 580–93, https://doi.org/10.7326/0003-4819-84-5-580.

Fricke, J., G. Avila, T. Keller et al., "Prevalence of Chronic Urticaria in Children and Adults Across the Globe: Systematic Review with Meta-Analysis," *Allergy: European Journal of Allergy and Clinical Immunology* 75, no. 2 (2020): 423–32, https://doi.org/10.1111/all.14037.

Greaves, M., "Chronic Urticaria," *Journal of Allergy and Clinical Immunology* 105, no. 4 (2000): 664–72, https://doi.org/10.1067/mai.2000.105706.

Guttman-Yassky, E., R. Bergman, C. Maor et al., "The Autologous Serum Skin Test in a Cohort of Chronic Idiopathic Urticaria Patients Compared to Respiratory Allergy Patients and Healthy Individuals," *Journal of the European Academy of Dermatology and Venereology* 21, no. 1 (2007): 35–39, https://doi.org/10.1111/j.1468-3083.2006.01852.x.

Katsarou-Katsari, A., M. Makris, E. Lagogianni et al., "Clinical Features and Natural History of Acquired Cold Urticaria in a Tertiary Referral Hospital: A 10-Year Prospective Study," *Journal of the European Academy of Dermatology and Venereology* 22, no. 12 (2008): 1405–11, https://doi.org/10.1111/j.1468-3083.2008.02840.x.

Kirby, J. D., C. N. Matthews, J. James et al., "The Incidence and Other Aspects of Factitious Wealing (Dermographism)," *British Journal of Dermatology* 85, no. 4 (1971): 331–35, https://doi.org/10.1111/j.1365-2133.1971.tb14027.x.

Kocaturk, E., M. Al-Ahmad, K. Krause et al., "Effects of Pregnancy on Chronic Urticaria: Results of the Preg-Cu Ucare Study," *Allergy: European Journal of Allergy and Clinical Immunology* 76, no. 10 (2021): 3133–44, https://doi.org/10.1111/all.14950.

Neittaanmaki, H., "Cold Urticaria. Clinical Findings in 220 Patients," *Journal of the American Academy of Dermatology* 13, no. 4 (1985): 636–44, https://doi.org/10.1016/s0190-9622(85)70208-3.

Orfan, N. A., and G. B. Kolski, "Physical Urticarias," *Annals of Allergy* 71, no. 3 (1993): 205–12, https://www.ncbi.nlm.nih.gov/pubmed/8372992.

Pappalardo, E., M. Cicardi, C. Duponchel et al., "Frequent De Novo Mutations and Exon Deletions in the C1 Inhibitor Gene of Patients with Angioedema," *Journal of Allergy and Clinical Immunology* 106, no. 6 (2000): 1147–54, https://doi.org/10.1067/mai.2000.110471.

Prosty, C., S. Gabrielli, P. Mule et al., "Cold Urticaria in a Pediatric Cohort: Clinical Characteristics, Management, and Natural History," *Pediatric Allergy and Immunology* 33, no. 3 (2022): e13751, https://doi.org/10.1111/pai.13751.

Rujitharanawong, C., K. Kulthanan, P. Tuchinda et al., "A Systematic Review of Aquagenic Urticaria-Subgroups and Treatment Options," *Journal of Allergy and Clinical Immunology: In Practice* 10, no. 8 (2022): 2154–62, https://doi.org/10.1016/j.jaip.2022.04.033.

Sabroe, R. A., C. E. Grattan, D. M. Francis et al., "The Autologous Serum Skin Test: A Screening Test for Autoantibodies in Chronic Idiopathic Urticaria," *British Journal of Dermatology* 140, no. 3 (1999): 446–52, https://doi.org/10.1046/j.1365-2133.1999.02707.x.

Sagonowsky, E., "The 20 Most Expensive Pharmacy Drugs in 2018, Featuring Names Big and Small," *Fierce Pharma*, January 1, 2025, https://www.fiercepharma.com/pharma/top-20-most-expensive-drugs-2018-featuring-names-big-and-small.

Sánchez, J., L. Alvarez, and R. Cardona, "Prospective Analysis of Clinical Evolution in Chronic Urticaria: Persistence, Remission, Recurrence, and Pruritus Alone," *World Allergy Organization Journal* 15, no. 10 (2022): 100705, https://doi.org/10.1016/j.waojou.2022.100705.

Terhorst-Molawi, D., L. Fox, F. Siebenhaar et al., "Stepping Down Treatment in Chronic Spontaneous Urticaria: What We Know and What We Don't Know," *American Journal of Clinical Dermatology* 24, no. 3 (2023): 397–404, https://doi.org/10.1007/s40257-023-00761-z.

Theoharides, T. C., "The Impact of Psychological Stress on Mast Cells," *Annals of Allergy, Asthma & Immunology* 125, no. 4 (2020): 388–92, https://doi.org/10.1016/j.anai.2020.07.007.

Zuraw, B. L., J. A. Bernstein, D. M. Lang et al., "A Focused Parameter Update: Hereditary Angioedema, Acquired C1 Inhibitor Deficiency, and Angiotensin-Converting Enzyme Inhibitor-Associated Angioedema," *Journal of Allergy and Clinical Immunology* 131, no. 6 (2013): 1491–93, https://doi.org/10.1016/j.jaci.2013.03.034.

Chapter 11—Asthma

Centers for Disease Control and Prevention, "About Underlying Cause of Death, 2018–2023, Single Race," CDC Wonder, accessed January 1, 2025, https://wonder.cdc.gov/ucd-icd10-expanded.html.

Al-Jahdali, H., A. Ahmed, A. Al-Harbi et al., "Improper Inhaler Technique Is Associated with Poor Asthma Control and Frequent Emergency Department Visits," *Allergy, Asthma & Clinical Immunology* 9, no. 1 (2013): 8, https://doi.org/10.1186/1710-1492-9-8.

Brenner, B., T. Corbridge, and A. Kazzi, "Intubation and Mechanical Ventilation of the Asthmatic Patient in Respiratory Failure," *Journal of Allergy and Clinical Immunology* 124, no. 2 Suppl. (2009): S19–28, https://doi.org/10.1016/j.jaci.2009.05.008.

Bronnimann, S., and B. Burrows, "A Prospective Study of the Natural History of Asthma: Remission and Relapse Rates," *Chest* 90, no. 4 (1986): 480–84, https://doi.org/10.1378/chest.90.4.480.

Cho-Reyes, S., B. R. Celli, C. Dembek et al., "Inhalation Technique Errors with Metered-Dose Inhalers Among Patients with Obstructive Lung Diseases: A Systematic Review and Meta-Analysis of U.S. Studies," *Chronic Obstructive Pulmonary Diseases* 6, no. 3 (2019): 267–80, https://doi.org/10.15326/jcopdf.6.3.2018.0168.

Christensen, P. M., J. H. Heimdal, K. L. Christopher et al., "ERS/ELS/ACCP 2013 International Consensus Conference Nomenclature on Inducible Laryngeal Obstructions," *European Respiratory Review* 24, no. 137 (2015): 445–50, https://doi.org/10.1183/16000617.0000 6513.

Cloutier, M. M., A. P. Baptist, K. V. Blake et al., "2020 Focused Updates to the Asthma Management Guidelines: A Report from the National Asthma Education and Prevention Program Coordinating Committee Expert Panel Working Group," *Journal of Allergy and Clinical Immunology* 146, no. 6 (2020): 1217–70, https://doi.org/10.1016 /j.jaci.2020.10.003.

Corlateanu, A., I. Stratan, S. Covantev et al., "Asthma and Stroke: A Narrative Review," *Asthma Research and Practice* 7, no. 1 (2021): 3, https://doi.org /10.1186/s40733-021-00069-x.

Ernst, P., B. Cai, L. Blais et al., "The Early Course of Newly Diagnosed Asthma," *American Journal of Medicine* 112, no. 1 (2002): 44–48, https://doi.org/10.1016/s0002-9343(01)01033-6.

Forrest, L. A., T. Husein, and O. Husein, "Paradoxical Vocal Cord Motion: Classification and Treatment," *Laryngoscope* 122, no. 4 (2012): 844–53, https://doi.org/10.1002/lary.23176.

Gonzalez, Marybel, "A Chicago Mother's Warning After Poor Air Quality Led to Her Daughter's Death," *CBS News*, accessed December 1, 2023, https://www.cbsnews.com/chicago/news/daughter-death-poor-air -quality/.

Gopallawa, I., R. Dehinwal, V. Bhatia et al., "A Four-Part Guide to Lung Immunology: Invasion, Inflammation, Immunity, and Intervention," *Frontiers in Immunology* 14 (2023): 1119564, https://doi.org/10.3389 /fimmu.2023.1119564.

Gruenwald, T., B. A. Seals, L. D. Knibbs et al., "Population Attributable Fraction of Gas Stoves and Childhood Asthma in the United States,"

Internatonal Journal of Environmental Research and Public Health 20, no. 1 (2022): https://doi.org/10.3390/ijerph20010075.

Kashtan, Y., M. Nicholson, C. J. Finnegan et al., "Nitrogen Dioxide Exposure, Health Outcomes, and Associated Demographic Disparities Due to Gas and Propane Combustion by U.S. Stoves," *Science Advances* 10, no. 18 (2024): eadm8680, https://doi.org/10.1126/sciadv.adm8680.

Kelly, H. W., A. L. Sternberg, R. Lescher et al., "Effect of Inhaled Glucocorticoids in Childhood on Adult Height," *New England Journal of Medicine* 367, no. 10 (2012): 904–12, https://doi.org/10.1056/NEJMoa1203229.

Kuruvilla, M. E., F. E. Lee, and G. B. Lee, "Understanding Asthma Phenotypes, Endotypes, and Mechanisms of Disease," *Clinical Reviews in Allergy & Immunology* 56, no. 2 (2019): 219–33, https://doi.org/10.1007/s12016-018-8712-1.

Levine, D., R. Respaut, K. Cooke et al., "A Son Died, His Parents Tried to Sue: How U.S. Courts Protect Big Pharma," Reuters, accessed November 1, 2023, https://www.reuters.com/investigates/special-report/usa-lawsuits-merck-singulair.

McArdle, C. E., T. C. Dowling, K. Carey et al., "Asthma-Associated Emergency Department Visits During the Canadian Wildfire Smoke Episodes—United States, April–August 2023," *MMWR Morbidity and Mortality Weekly Report* 72, no. 34 (2023): 926–32, https://doi.org/10.15585/mmwr.mm7234a5.

Millard, M., M. Hart, and S. Barnes, "Validation of Rules of Two as a Paradigm for Assessing Asthma Control," *Baylor University Medical Center Proceedings* 27, no. 2 (2014): 79–82, https://doi.org/10.1080/08998280.2014.11929063.

Pessôa, C. L. C., M. J. D. S. Mattos, A. R. M. Alho et al., "Most Frequent Errors in Inhalation Technique of Patients with Asthma Treated at a Tertiary Care Hospital," *Einstein (São Paulo)* 17, no. 2 (2019): eAO4397, https://doi.org/10.31744/einstein_journal/2019AO4397.

Peterson, J. W., and Y. M. Sterling, "Children's Perceptions of Asthma: African American Children Use Metaphors to Make Sense of Asthma," *Journal of Pediatric Health Care* 23, no. 2 (2009): 93–100, https://doi.org/10.1016/j.pedhc.2007.10.002.

Weiss, L. N., "The Diagnosis of Wheezing in Children," *American Family Physician* 77, no. 8 (2008): 1109–14, https://www.ncbi.nlm.nih.gov/pubmed/18481558.

Chapter 12—Anaphylaxis

Beaudouin, E., J. M. Renaudin, M. Morisset et al., "Food-Dependent Exercise-Induced Anaphylaxis—Update and Current Data," *European Annals of Allergy and Clinical Immunology* 38, no. 2 (2006): 45–51, https://www.ncbi.nlm.nih.gov/pubmed/16711535.

Behzadi, A. H., Y. Zhao, Z. Farooq et al., "Immediate Allergic Reactions to Gadolinium-Based Contrast Agents: A Systematic Review and Meta-Analysis," *Radiology* 286, no. 2 (2018): 731, https://doi.org/10.1148/radiol.2017174037.

Bush, W. H., and D. P. Swanson, "Acute Reactions to Intravascular Contrast Media: Types, Risk Factors, Recognition, and Specific Treatment," *American Journal of Roentgenology* 157, no. 6 (1991): 1153–61, https://doi.org/10.2214/ajr.157.6.1950858.

Golden, D. B. K., J. Demain, T. Freeman et al., "Stinging Insect Hypersensitivity: A Practice Parameter Update 2016," *Annals of Allergy, Asthma & Immunology* 118, no. 1 (2017): 28–54, https://doi.org/10.1016/j.anai.2016.10.031.

Golden, D. B. K., J. Wang, S. Waserman et al., "Anaphylaxis: A 2023 Practice Parameter Update," *Annals of Allergy, Asthma & Immunology* 132, no. 2 (2024): 124–76, https://doi.org/10.1016/j.anai.2023.09.015.

Habib, M. A. H., and M. N. Ismail, "Hevea Brasiliensis Latex Proteomics: A Review of Analytical Methods and the Way Forward," *Journal of Plant Research* 134, no. 1 (2021): 43–53, https://doi.org/10.1007/s10265-020-01231-x.

Hamann, C. P., and S. A. Kick, "Allergies Associated with Medical Gloves: Manufacturing Issues," *Dermatologic Clinics* 12, no. 3 (1994): 547–59, https://www.ncbi.nlm.nih.gov/pubmed/7923952.

Iribarren, C., I. V. Tolstykh, M. K. Miller et al., "Asthma and the Prospective Risk of Anaphylactic Shock and Other Allergy Diagnoses in a Large Integrated Health Care Delivery System," *Annals of Allergy, Asthma & Immunology* 104, no. 5 (2010): 371–77, https://doi.org/10.1016/j.anai.2010.03.004.

Jacob, J. L., J. d'Auzac, and J. C. Prevôt, "The Composition of Natural Latex from Hevea Brasiliensis," *Clinical Reviews in Allergy & Immunology* 11, no. 3 (1993): 325–37, https://doi.org/10.1007/BF02914415.

Kekwick, R. G., "The Modification of Polypeptides in Hevea Brasiliensis Latex Resulting from Storage and Processing," *Clinical Reviews in Allergy &*

Immunology 11, no. 3 (1993): 339–53, https://doi.org/10.1007
/BF02914416.

Kelly, K. J., and G. Sussman, "Latex Allergy: Where Are We Now and
How Did We Get There?" *Journal of Allergy and Clinical Immunology: In
Practice* 5, no. 5 (2017): 1212–16, https://doi.org/10.1016/j.jaip.2017
.05.029.

Kliff, Sarah, "EpiPen's 400 Percent Price Hike Tells Us a Lot About
What's Wrong with American Health Care," *Vox*, accessed October 4,
2024, https://www.vox.com/2016/8/23/12608316/epipen-price
-mylan.

Mari, A., E. Scala, C. D'Ambrosio et al., "Latex Allergy Within a Cohort of
Not-at-Risk Subjects with Respiratory Symptoms: Prevalence of Latex
Sensitization and Assessment of Diagnostic Tools," *International Archives
of Allergy and Immunology* 143, no. 2 (2007): 135–43, https://doi.org
/10.1159/000099080.

Motosue, M. S., M. F. Bellolio, H. K. Van Houten et al., "Increasing
Emergency Department Visits for Anaphylaxis, 2005–2014," *Journal of
Allergy and Clinical Immunology: In Practice* 5, no. 1 (2017): 171–75 e3,
https://doi.org/10.1016/j.jaip.2016.08.013.

Neugut, A. I., A. T. Ghatak, and R. L. Miller, "Anaphylaxis in the United
States: An Investigation into Its Epidemiology," *Archives of Internal
Medicine* 161, no. 1 (2001): 15–21, https://doi.org/10.1001/archinte
.161.1.15.

Pumphrey, R. S., "Fatal Anaphylaxis in the UK, 1992–2001," *Novartis
Foundation Symposium* 257 (2004): 116–28; discussion 128–32,
157–60, 276–85, https://www.ncbi.nlm.nih.gov/pubmed/1502
5395.

Romano, A., M. Di Fonso, F. Giuffreda et al., "Food-Dependent Exercise-
Induced Anaphylaxis: Clinical and Laboratory Findings in 54 Subjects,"
International Archives of Allergy and Immunology 125, no. 3 (2001):
264–72, https://doi.org/10.1159/000053825.

Scott, Dylan, "Can We Solve the EpiPen Cost Crisis?" *Vox*, accessed
September 20, 2024, https://www.vox.com/policy/23658275/epipen
-cost-price-how-much.

Simons, F. E., L. R. Ardusso, M. B. Bilo et al., "World Allergy Organization
Anaphylaxis Guidelines: Summary," *Journal of Allergy and Clinical
Immunology* 127, no. 3 (2011): 587–93 e1–22, https://doi.org/10.1016
/j.jaci.2011.01.038.

Summers, C. W., R. S. Pumphrey, C. N. Woods et al., "Factors Predicting Anaphylaxis to Peanuts and Tree Nuts in Patients Referred to a Specialist Center," *Journal of Allergy and Clinical Immunology* 121, no. 3 (2008): 632–38 e2, https://doi.org/10.1016/j.jaci.2007.12.003.

Tejedor Alonso, M. A., M. Moro Moro, and M. V. Mûgica García, "Epidemiology of Anaphylaxis," *Clinical and Experimental Allergy* 45, no. 6 (2015): 1027–39, https://doi.org/10.1111/cea.12418.

Thompson, J. M., A. Carpenter, G. J. Kersh et al., "Geographic Distribution of Suspected Alpha-Gal Syndrome Cases—United States, January 2017–December 2022," *MMWR Morbidity and Mortality Weekly Report* 72, no. 30 (2023): 815–20, https://doi.org/10.15585/mmwr.mm7230a2.

Triggiani, M., V. Patella, R. I. Staiano et al., "Allergy and the Cardiovascular System," *Clinical and Experimental Immunology* 153, no. 1 Suppl. (2008): 7–11, https://doi.org/10.1111/j.1365-2249.2008.03714.x.

Truscott, W., and L. Roley, "Glove-Associated Reactions: Addressing an Increasing Concern," *Dermatology Nursing* 7, no. 5 (1995): 283–90, 303, quiz 291–92, https://www.ncbi.nlm.nih.gov/pubmed/869 5318.

Wolfson, A. R., D. Wong, E. M. Abrams et al., "Diphenhydramine: Time to Move On?" *Journal of Allergy and Clinical Immunology: In Practice* 10, no. 12 (2022): 3124–30, https://doi.org/10.1016/j.jaip.2022.07.018.

Wood, R. A., C. A. Camargo Jr., P. Lieberman et al., "Anaphylaxis in America: The Prevalence and Characteristics of Anaphylaxis in the United States," *Journal of Allergy and Clinical Immunology* 133, no. 2 (2014): 461–67, https://doi.org/10.1016/j.jaci.2013.08.016.

Zilberstein, J., M. T. McCurdy, and M. E. Winters, "Anaphylaxis," *Journal of Emergency Medicine* 47, no. 2 (2014): 182–87, https://doi.org/10.1016/j.jemermed.2014.04.018.

Chapter 13—Medication and Vaccine Allergies

"Lightning Victims," National Weather Service, accessed October 4, 2024, https://www.weather.gov/safety/lightning-victims.

Banerji, A., P. G. Wickner, R. Saff et al., "mRNA Vaccines to Prevent Covid-19 Disease and Reported Allergic Reactions: Current Evidence and Suggested Approach," *Journal of Allergy and Clinical Immunology: In Practice* 9, no. 4 (2021): 1423–37, https://doi.org/10.1016/j.jaip.2020.12.047.

Bastuji-Garin, S., B. Rzany, R. S. Stern et al., "Clinical Classification of Cases of Toxic Epidermal Necrolysis, Stevens-Johnson Syndrome, and Erythema Multiforme," *Archives of Dermatology* 129, no. 1 (1993): 92–96, https://www.ncbi.nlm.nih.gov/pubmed/8420497.

Blanca, M., M. J. Torres, J. J. Garcia et al., "Natural Evolution of Skin Test Sensitivity in Patients Allergic to Beta-Lactam Antibiotics," *Journal of Allergy and Clinical Immunology* 103, no. 5 (1999): 918–24, https://doi.org/10.1016/s0091-6749(99)70439-2.

Blumenthal, K. G., N. Lu, Y. Zhang et al., "Recorded Penicillin Allergy and Risk of Mortality: A Population-Based Matched Cohort Study," *Journal of General Internal Medicine* 34, no. 9 (2019): 1685–87, https://doi.org/10.1007/s11606-019-04991-y.

Bohlke, K., R. L. Davis, S. M. Marcy et al., "Risk of Anaphylaxis After Vaccination of Children and Adolescents," *Pediatrics* 112, no. 4 (2003): 815–20, https://doi.org/10.1542/peds.112.4.815.

Chaby, G., C. Maldini, C. Haddad et al., "Incidence of and Mortality from Epidermal Necrolysis (Stevens-Johnson Syndrome/Toxic Epidermal Necrolysis) in France During 2003–16: A Four-Source Capture-Recapture Estimate," *British Journal of Dermatology* 182, no. 3 (2020): 618–24, https://doi.org/10.1111/bjd.18424.

Choe, Y. J., H. Lee, J. H. Kim et al., "Anaphylaxis Following Vaccination Among Children in Asia: A Large-Linked Database Study," *Allergy: European Journal of Allergy and Clinical Immunology* 76, no. 4 (2021): 1246–49, https://doi.org/10.1111/all.14562.

Davies, D. M., ed., *Textbook of Adverse Drug Reactions*, 4th ed. (Oxford: Oxford University Press, 1991).

Devchand, M., and J. A. Trubiano, "Penicillin Allergy: A Practical Approach to Assessment and Prescribing," *Australian Prescriber* 42, no. 6 (2019): 192–99, https://doi.org/10.18773/austprescr.2019.065.

Fernandez-Nieto, D., J. Hammerle, M. Fernandez-Escribano et al., "Skin Manifestations of the BNT162b2 mRNA COVID-19 Vaccine in Healthcare Workers. 'COVID-Arm': A Clinical and Histological Characterization," *Journal of the European Academy of Dermatology and Venereology* 35, no. 7 (2021): e425–27, https://doi.org/10.1111/jdv.17250.

Greenhawt, M., T. E. Dribin, E. M. Abrams et al., "Updated Guidance Regarding the Risk of Allergic Reactions to COVID-19 Vaccines and

Recommended Evaluation and Management: A GRADE Assessment and International Consensus Approach," *Journal of Allergy and Clinical Immunology* 152, no. 2 (2023): 309–25, https://doi.org/10.1016/j.jaci.2023.05.019.

Hsu, D. Y., J. Brieva, N. B. Silverberg et al., "Morbidity and Mortality of Stevens-Johnson Syndrome and Toxic Epidermal Necrolysis in United States Adults," *Journal of Investigative Dermatology* 136, no. 7 (2016): 1387–97, https://doi.org/10.1016/j.jid.2016.03.023.

Jaggers, J., and A. R. Wolfson, "mRNA COVID-19 Vaccine Anaphylaxis: Epidemiology, Risk Factors, and Evaluation," *Current Allergy and Asthma Reports* 23, no. 3 (2023): 195–200, https://doi.org/10.1007/s11882-023-01065-2.

Kardaun, S. H., P. Sekula, L. Valeyrie-Allanore et al., "Drug Reaction with Eosinophilia and Systemic Symptoms (DRESS): An Original Multisystem Adverse Drug Reaction. Results from the Prospective Regiscar Study," *British Journal of Dermatology* 169, no. 5 (2013): 1071–80, https://doi.org/10.1111/bjd.12501.

Khan, D. A., A. Banerji, K. G. Blumenthal et al., "Drug Allergy: A 2022 Practice Parameter Update," *Journal of Allergy and Clinical Immunology* 150, no. 6 (2022): 1333–93, https://doi.org/10.1016/j.jaci.2022.08.028.

Klein, N. P., N. Lewis, K. Goddard et al., "Surveillance for Adverse Events After COVID-19 mRNA Vaccination," *JAMA* 326, no. 14 (2021): 1390–99, https://doi.org/10.1001/jama.2021.15072.

Klimek, L., N. Novak, B. Cabanillas et al., "Allergenic Components of the mRNA-1273 Vaccine for COVID-19: Possible Involvement of Polyethylene Glycol and IgG-Mediated Complement Activation," *Allergy: European Journal of Allergy and Clinical Immunology* 76, no. 11 (2021): 3307–13, https://doi.org/10.1111/all.14794.

Lawley, T. J., L. Bielory, P. Gascon et al., "A Prospective Clinical and Immunologic Analysis of Patients with Serum Sickness," *New England Journal of Medicine* 311, no. 22 (1984): 1407–13, https://doi.org/10.1056/NEJM198411293112204.

Patterson, R. A., and H. A. Stankewicz, eds., *Penicillin Allergy* (StatPearls Publishing, 2025).

Sassolas, B., C. Haddad, M. Mockenhaupt et al., "ALDEN, an Algorithm for Assessment of Drug Causality in Stevens-Johnson Syndrome and Toxic Epidermal Necrolysis: Comparison with Case-Control Analysis," *Clinical*

Pharmacology and Therapeutics 88, no. 1 (2010): 60–68, https://doi.org/10.1038/clpt.2009.252.

Shenoy, E. S., E. Macy, T. Rowe et al., "Evaluation and Management of Penicillin Allergy: A Review," *JAMA* 321, no. 2 (2019): 188–99, https://doi.org/10.1001/jama.2018.19283.

Su, C., A. Belmont, J. Liao et al., "Evaluating the Pen-Fast Clinical Decision-Making Tool to Enhance Penicillin Allergy Delabeling," *JAMA Internal Medicine* 183, no. 8 (2023): 883–85, https://doi.org/10.1001/jamainternmed.2023.1572.

Su, J. R., P. L. Moro, C. S. Ng et al., "Anaphylaxis After Vaccination Reported to the Vaccine Adverse Event Reporting System, 1990–2016," *Journal of Allergy and Clinical Immunology* 143, no. 4 (2019): 1465–73, https://doi.org/10.1016/j.jaci.2018.12.1003.

Ushigome, Y., Y. Kano, T. Ishida et al., "Short- and Long-Term Outcomes of 34 Patients with Drug-Induced Hypersensitivity Syndrome in a Single Institution," *Journal of the American Academy of Dermatology* 68, no. 5 (2013): 721–28, https://doi.org/10.1016/j.jaad.2012.10.017.

Washrawirul, C., J. Triwatcharikorn, J. Phannajit et al., "Global Prevalence and Clinical Manifestations of Cutaneous Adverse Reactions Following COVID-19 Vaccination: A Systematic Review and Meta-Analysis," *Journal of the European Academy of Dermatology and Venereology* 36, no. 11 (2022): 1947–68, https://doi.org/10.1111/jdv.18294.

Wolfson, A. R., L. Zhou, Y. Li et al., "Drug Reaction with Eosinophilia and Systemic Symptoms (DRESS) Syndrome Identified in the Electronic Health Record Allergy Module," *Journal of Allergy and Clinical Immunology: In Practice* 7, no. 2 (2019): 633–40, https://doi.org/10.1016/j.jaip.2018.08.013.

Chapter 14—Mast Cell Disorders

Akin, C., "Mast Cell Activation Syndromes," *Journal of Allergy and Clinical Immunology* 140, no. 2 (2017): 349–55, https://doi.org/10.1016/j.jaci.2017.06.007.

Bonadonna, P., M. Pagani, W. Aberer et al., "Drug Hypersensitivity in Clonal Mast Cell Disorders: ENDA/EAACI Position Paper," *Allergy: European Journal of Allergy and Clinical Immunology* 70, no. 7 (2015): 755–63, https://doi.org/10.1111/all.12617.

Bonamichi-Santos, R., K. Yoshimi-Kanamori, P. Giavina-Bianchi et al., "Association of Postural Tachycardia Syndrome and Ehlers-Danlos

Syndrome with Mast Cell Activation Disorders," *Immunology and Allergy Clinics of North America* 38, no. 3 (2018): 497–504, https://doi.org/10.1016/j.iac.2018.04.004.

Buttgereit, T., S. Gu, L. Carneiro-Leao et al., "Idiopathic Mast Cell Activation Syndrome Is More Often Suspected Than Diagnosed—A Prospective Real-Life Study," *Allergy: European Journal of Allergy and Clinical Immunology* 77, no. 9 (2022): 2794–802, https://doi.org/10.1111/all.15304.

Castells, M., and J. Butterfield, "Mast Cell Activation Syndrome and Mastocytosis: Initial Treatment Options and Long-Term Management," *Journal of Allergy and Clinical Immunology: In Practice* 7, no. 4 (2019): 1097–106, https://doi.org/10.1016/j.jaip.2019.02.002.

Castells, M., M. P. Giannetti, M. J. Hamilton et al., "Mast Cell Activation Syndrome: Current Understanding and Research Needs," *Journal of Allergy and Clinical Immunology* 154, no. 2 (2024): 255–63, https://doi.org/10.1016/j.jaci.2024.05.025.

Galli, S. J., "The Mast Cell-IgE Paradox: From Homeostasis to Anaphylaxis," *American Journal of Pathology* 186, no. 2 (2016): 212–24, https://doi.org/10.1016/j.ajpath.2015.07.025.

Hartmann, K., L. Escribano, C. Grattan et al., "Cutaneous Manifestations in Patients with Mastocytosis: Consensus Report of the European Competence Network on Mastocytosis; the American Academy of Allergy, Asthma & Immunology; and the European Academy of Allergology and Clinical Immunology," *Journal of Allergy and Clinical Immunology* 137, no. 1 (2016): 35–45, https://doi.org/10.1016/j.jaci.2015.08.034.

Huang, J., J. C. Del Valle, and A. White, "The Prevalence of Hereditary Alpha-Tryptasemia in Patients Diagnosed with POTS via Tilt Table Testing," *Journal of Allergy and Clinical Immunology* 147, no. 2 (2021), https://doi.org/10.1016/j.jaci.2020.12.492.

Ishikawa, T., T. Shimada, N. Kessoku et al., "Inhibition of Rat Mast Cell Degranulation and Histamine Release by Histamine-Rat Gammaglobulin Conjugate," *International Archives of Allergy and Applied Immunology* 59, no. 4 (1979): 403–7, https://doi.org/10.1159/000232287.

Konnikova, L., T. O. Robinson, A. H. Owings et al., "Small Intestinal Immunopathology and GI-Associated Antibody Formation in Hereditary

Alpha-Tryptasemia," *Journal of Allergy and Clinical Immunology* 148, no. 3 (2021): 813–21 e7, https://doi.org/10.1016/j.jaci .2021.04.004.

Lyons, J. J., "Inherited and Acquired Determinants of Serum Tryptase Levels in Humans," *Annals of Allergy, Asthma & Immunology* 127, no. 4 (2021): 420–26, https://doi.org/10.1016/j.anai.2021.06.019.

Maddur, M. S., S. V. Kaveri, and J. Bayry, "Circulating Normal IgG as Stimulator of Regulatory T Cells: Lessons from Intravenous Immunoglobulin," *Trends in Immunology* 38, no. 11 (2017): 789–92, https://doi.org/10.1016/j.it.2017.08.008.

McLaughlin, P. J., D. P. McHugh, M. J. Magister et al., "Endogenous Opioid Inhibition of Proliferation of T and B Cell Subpopulations in Response to Immunization for Experimental Autoimmune Encephalomyelitis," *BMC Immunology* 16, no. 1: 24 (2015), https://doi.org/10.1186/s12865-015 -0093-0.

Moodley, I., and J. L. Mongar, "IgG Receptors on the Mast Cell," *Agents and Actions* 11, no. 1–2 (1981): 77–83, https://doi.org/10.1007/BF019 91464.

Parente, R., V. Giudice, C. Cardamone et al., "Secretory and Membrane-Associated Biomarkers of Mast Cell Activation and Proliferation," *International Journal of Molecular Sciences* 24, no. 8 (2023), https://doi.org/10.3390/ijms24087071.

Solomon, B. D., and P. Khatri, "Clustering of Clinical Symptoms Using Large Language Models Reveals Low Diagnostic Specificity of Proposed Alternatives to Consensus Mast Cell Activation Syndrome Criteria," *Journal of Allergy and Clinical Immunology* 155, no. 1 (2025): 213–18 e4, https://doi.org/10.1016/j.jaci.2024.09.006.

Theoharides, T. C., P. Valent, and C. Akin, "Mast Cells, Mastocytosis, and Related Disorders," *New England Journal of Medicine* 373, no. 2 (2015): 163–72, https://doi.org/10.1056/NEJMra1409760.

Valent, P., C. Akin, K. Hartmann et al., "Updated Diagnostic Criteria and Classification of Mast Cell Disorders: A Consensus Proposal," *HemaSphere* 5, no. 11 (2021): e646, https://doi.org/10.1097/HS9 .0000000000000646.

Valent, P., C. Akin, P. Bonadonna et al., "Proposed Diagnostic Algorithm for Patients with Suspected Mast Cell Activation Syndrome," *Journal of Allergy and Clinical Immunology: In Practice* 7, no. 4 (2019): 1125–33 e1, https://doi.org/10.1016/j.jaip.2019.01.006.

Vazquez, M., J. Chovanec, J. Kim et al., "Hereditary Alpha-Tryptasemia Modifies Clinical Phenotypes Among Individuals with Congenital Hypermobility Disorders," *Human Genetics and Genomics Advances* 3, no. 2 (2022): 100094, https://doi.org/10.1016/j.xhgg.2022.100094.

Weiler, C. R., K. F. Austen, C. Akin et al., "AAAAI Mast Cell Disorders Committee Work Group Report: Mast Cell Activation Syndrome (MCAS) Diagnosis and Management," *Journal of Allergy and Clinical Immunology* 144, no. 4 (2019): 883–96, https://doi.org/10.1016/j.jaci .2019.08.023.

Weinstock, L. B., J. B. Brook, T. L. Myers et al., "Successful Treatment of Postural Orthostatic Tachycardia and Mast Cell Activation Syndromes Using Naltrexone, Immunoglobulin and Antibiotic Treatment," *BMJ Case Reports* 2018, https://doi.org/10.1136/bcr-2017-221405.

Zaghmout, T., L. Maclachlan, N. Bedi et al., "Low Prevalence of Idiopathic Mast Cell Activation Syndrome Among 703 Patients with Suspected Mast Cell Disorders," *Journal of Allergy and Clinical Immunology: In Practice* 12, no. 3 (2024): 753–61, https://doi.org/10.1016/j.jaip .2023.11.041.

Chapter 15—Over-the-Counter and Prescription Medications

Federal Aviation Administration, "Allergy—Antihistamine & Immunotherapy Medication," updated October 26, 2022, accessed November 2, 2024, https://www.faa.gov/ame_guide/media/Allergy AntihistamineImmunotherapyMedication.pdf.

U.S. Food and Drug Administration, "FDA Warns About Serious Problems with High Doses of the Allergy Medicine Diphenhydramine (Benadryl)," FDA Drug Safety Communication, September 24, 2020, accessed September 24, 2024, https://www.fda.gov/drugs/drug-safety -and-availability/fda-warns-about-serious-problems-high-doses -allergy-medicine-diphenhydramine-benadryl.

Agostini, J. V., L. S. Leo-Summers, and S. K. Inouye, "Cognitive and Other Adverse Effects of Diphenhydramine Use in Hospitalized Older Patients," *Archives of Internal Medicine* 161, no. 17 (2001): 2091–97, https://doi .org/10.1001/archinte.161.17.2091.

Boyle, J., M. Eriksson, N. Stanley et al., "Allergy Medication in Japanese Volunteers: Treatment Effect of Single Doses on Nocturnal Sleep Architecture and Next Day Residual Effects," *Current Medical Research and Opinion* 22, no. 7 (2006): 1343–51, https://doi.org/10 .1185/030079906X112660.

Breneman, D. L., "Cetirizine Versus Hydroxyzine and Placebo in Chronic Idiopathic Urticaria," *Annals of Pharmacotherapy* 30, no. 10 (1996): 1075–79, https://doi.org/10.1177/106002809603001001.

de Leon, J., and D. M. Nikoloff, "Paradoxical Excitation on Diphenhydramine May Be Associated with Being a CYP2D6 Ultrarapid Metabolizer: Three Case Reports," *CNS Spectrums* 13, no. 2 (2008): 133–35, https://doi.org /10.1017/s109285290001628x.

Dinwiddie, A. T., L. J. Tanz, and J. Bitting, "Notes from the Field: Antihistamine Positivity and Involvement in Drug Overdose Deaths—44 Jurisdictions, United States, 2019–2020," *MMWR Morbidity and Mortality Weekly Report* 71, no. 41 (2022): 1308–10, https://doi.org/10 .15585/mmwr.mm7141a4.

Dykewicz, M. S., D. V. Wallace, D. J. Amrol et al., "Rhinitis 2020: A Practice Parameter Update," *Journal of Allergy and Clinical Immunology* 146, no. 4 (2020): 721–67, https://doi.org/10.1016/j.jaci.2020.07.007.

Ekhart, C., P. van der Horst, and F. van Hunsel, "Unbearable Pruritus After Withdrawal of (Levo) Cetirizine," *Drug Safety—Case Reports* 3, no. 1 (2016): 16, https://doi.org/10.1007/s40800-016-0041-9.

Emanuel, M. B., "Histamine and the Antiallergic Antihistamines: A History of Their Discoveries," *Clinical and Experimental Allergy* 29, no. 3 Suppl. (1999): 1–11; discussion 12, https://doi.org/10.1046/j .1365-2222.1999.00004.x-i1.

Graf, P. M., and H. Hallen, "One Year Follow-up of Patients with Rhinitis Medicamentosa After Vasoconstrictor Withdrawal," *American Journal of Rhinology & Allergy* 11, no. 1 (1997): 67–72, https://doi.org/10 .2500/105065897781446865.

Hatton, R. C., and L. Hendeles, "Why Is Oral Phenylephrine on the Market After Compelling Evidence of Its Ineffectiveness as a Decongestant?" *Annals of Pharmacotherapy* 56, no. 11 (2022): 1275–78, https://doi.org/10.1177/10600280221081526.

Iseric, E., and J. C. Verster, "The Common Cold: The Need for an Effective Treatment amid the FDA Discussion on Oral Phenylephrine," *Journal of Allergy and Clinical Immunology: Global* 3, no. 4 (2024): 100318, https:// doi.org/10.1016/j.jacig.2024.100318.

Lee, L. A., R. Sterling, J. Maspero et al., "Growth Velocity Reduced with Once-Daily Fluticasone Furoate Nasal Spray in Prepubescent Children with Perennial Allergic Rhinitis," *Journal of Allergy and Clinical*

Immunology: In Practice 2, no. 4 (2014): 421–27, https://doi.org/10
.1016/j.jaip.2014.04.008.

Nicholson, A. N., B. M. Stone, C. Turner et al., "Antihistamines and Aircrew:
Usefulness of Fexofenadine," *Aviation, Space, and Environmental Medicine*
71, no. 1 (2000): 2–6, https://www.ncbi.nlm
.nih.gov/pubmed/10632124.

Park, J. H., J. H. Godbold, D. Chung et al., "Comparison of Cetirizine and
Diphenhydramine in the Treatment of Acute Food-Induced Allergic
Reactions," *Journal of Allergy and Clinical Immunology* 128, no. 5 (2011):
1127–28, https://doi.org/10.1016/j.jaci.2011.08.026.

Pitsios, C., D. Papadopoulos, E. Kompoti et al., "Efficacy and Safety of
Mometasone Furoate vs Nedocromil Sodium as Prophylactic Treatment
for Moderate/Severe Seasonal Allergic Rhinitis," *Annals of Allergy,
Asthma & Immunology* 96, no. 5 (2006): 673–78, https://doi.org/10.1016
/S1081-1206(10)61064-2.

Ratliff, J. C., J. A. Barber, L. B. Palmese et al., "Association of
Prescription H1 Antihistamine Use with Obesity: Results from the
National Health and Nutrition Examination Survey," *Obesity (Silver
Spring)* 18, no. 12 (2010): 2398–400, https://doi.org/10.1038
/oby.2010.176.

Sakata, T., H. Yoshimatsu, and M. Kurokawa, "Hypothalamic Neuronal
Histamine: Implications of Its Homeostatic Control of Energy
Metabolism," *Nutrition* 13, no. 5 (1997): 403–11, https://doi.org/10
.1016/s0899-9007(97)91277-6.

Sateia, M. J., D. J. Buysse, A. D. Krystal et al., "Clinical Practice Guideline for
the Pharmacologic Treatment of Chronic Insomnia in Adults: An
American Academy of Sleep Medicine Clinical Practice Guideline," *Journal
of Clinical Sleep Medicine* 13, no. 2 (2017): 307–49, https://doi
.org/10.5664/jcsm.6470.

Simons, F. E., J. L. McMillan, and K. J. Simons, "A Double-Blind, Single-Dose,
Crossover Comparison of Cetirizine, Terfenadine, Loratadine, Astemizole,
and Chlorpheniramine Versus Placebo: Suppressive Effects on Histamine-
Induced Wheals and Flares During 24 Hours in Normal Subjects," *Journal
of Allergy and Clinical Immunology* 86, no. 4, Pt. 1 (1990): 540–47,
https://www.ncbi.nlm.nih.gov/pubmed/1977781.

Tashiro, M., X. Duan, M. Kato et al., "Brain Histamine H_1 Receptor
Occupancy of Orally Administered Antihistamines, Bepotastine and

Diphenhydramine, Measured by PET with 11C-Doxepin," *British Journal of Clinical Pharmacology* 65, no. 6 (2008): 811–21, https://doi .org/10.1111/j.1365-2125.2008.03143.x.

Thakkar, M. M., "Histamine in the Regulation of Wakefulness," *Sleep Medicine Reviews* 15, no. 1 (2011): 65–74, https://doi.org/10.1016/j .smrv.2010.06.004.

Vaidyanathan, S., P. Williamson, K. Clearie et al., "Fluticasone Reverses Oxymetazoline-Induced Tachyphylaxis of Response and Rebound Congestion," *American Journal of Respiratory and Critical Care Medicine* 182, no. 1 (2010): 19–24, https://doi.org/10.1164/rccm .200911-1701OC.

Vuurman, E. F., L. M. van Veggel, R. L. Sanders et al., "Effects of Semprex-D and Diphenhydramine on Learning in Young Adults with Seasonal Allergic Rhinitis," *Annals of Allergy, Asthma & Immunology* 76, no. 3 (1996): 247–52, https://doi.org/10.1016/S1081-1206(10)63435-7.

Weiler, J. M., J. R. Bloomfield, G. G. Woodworth et al., "Effects of Fexofenadine, Diphenhydramine, and Alcohol on Driving Performance: A Randomized, Placebo-Controlled Trial in the Iowa Driving Simulator," *Annals of Internal Medicine* 132, no. 5 (2000): 354–63, https://doi.org /10.7326/0003-4819-132-5-200003070-00004.

Wolfson, A. R., D. Wong, E. M. Abrams et al., "Diphenhydramine: Time to Move On?" *Journal of Allergy and Clinical Immunology: In Practice* 10, no. 12 (2022): 3124–30, https://doi.org/10.1016/j.jaip.2022.07.018.

Chapter 16—Immunotherapy

"Study in Pediatric Subjects with Peanut Allergy to Evaluate Efficacy and Safety of Dupilumab as Adjunct to AR101 (Peanut Oral Immunotherapy)," National Library of Medicine, accessed December 2, 2024, https:// clinicaltrials.gov/study/NCT03682770.

Abramson, M. J., R. M. Puy, and J. M. Weiner, "Injection Allergen Immunotherapy for Asthma," *Cochrane Database of Systematic Reviews* 8 (2010): CD001186, https://doi.org/10.1002/14651858 .CD001186.pub2.

Akdis, M., and C. A. Akdis, "Mechanisms of Allergen-Specific Immunotherapy: Multiple Suppressor Factors at Work in Immune Tolerance to Allergens," *Journal of Allergy and Clinical Immunology* 133, no. 3 (2014): 621–31, https://doi.org/10.1016/j.jaci.2013.12.1088.

Allam, J. P., and N. Novak, "Immunological Mechanisms of Sublingual Immunotherapy," *Current Opinion in Allergy and Clinical Immunology* 14, no. 6 (2014): 564–69, https://doi.org/10.1097/ACI.0000000000000118.

Andorf, S., N. Purington, W. M. Block et al., "Anti-IgE Treatment with Oral Immunotherapy in Multifood Allergic Participants: A Double-Blind, Randomised, Controlled Trial," *Lancet Gastroenterology & Hepatology* 3, no. 2 (2018): 85–94, https://doi.org/10.1016/S2468 -1253(17)30392-8.

Begin, P., E. S. Chan, H. Kim et al., "CSACI Guidelines for the Ethical, Evidence-Based and Patient-Oriented Clinical Practice of Oral Immunotherapy in IgE-Mediated Food Allergy," *Allergy, Asthma & Clinical Immunology* 16 (2020): 20, https://doi.org/10.1186/s13223 -020-0413-7.

Begin, P., T. Dominguez, S. P. Wilson et al., "Phase 1 Results of Safety and Tolerability in a Rush Oral Immunotherapy Protocol to Multiple Foods Using Omalizumab," *Allergy, Asthma & Clinical Immunology* 10, no. 1 (2014): 7, https://doi.org/10.1186/1710-1492-10-7.

Berger, W. E., N. Faris, M. Weinstein et al., "Randomized, Placebo-Controlled, Phase 1 Safety Study of Oral Mucosal Immunotherapy in Peanut Allergic Adults," *Annals of Allergy, Asthma & Immunology* 134, no. 4 (2025): 448–56, https://doi.org/10.1016/j.anai.2025.01.013.

Blessing, M. H., and D. M. Reiner, "Studies on Chromoproteins of Cardiac and Skeletal Muscle of Caimans (*Caiman sclerops*)," *Pflügers Archiv—European Journal of Physiology* 361, no. 1 (1975): 101–3, https://doi.org/10.1007/BF00587349.

Chinthrajah, R. S., N. Purington, S. Andorf et al., "Sustained Outcomes in Oral Immunotherapy for Peanut Allergy (Poised Study): A Large, Randomised, Double-Blind, Placebo-Controlled, Phase 2 Study," *The Lancet* 394, no. 10207 (2019): 1437–49, https://doi.org/10.1016/S0140 -6736(19)31793-3.

Chu, D. K., R. A. Wood, S. French et al., "Oral Immunotherapy for Peanut Allergy (PACE): A Systematic Review and Meta-Analysis of Efficacy and Safety," *The Lancet* 393, no. 10187 (2019): 2222–32, https://doi .org/10.1016/S0140-6736(19)30420-9.

Cox, L., H. Nelson, R. Lockey et al., "Allergen Immunotherapy: A Practice Parameter Third Update," *Journal of Allergy and Clinical Immunology* 127, no. 1 Suppl. (2011): S1–55, https://doi.org/10.1016/j.jaci.2010 .09.034.

Du Toit, G., K. R. Brown, A. Vereda et al., "Oral Immunotherapy for Peanut Allergy in Children 1 to Less Than 4 Years of Age," *New England Journal of Medicine: Evidence* 2, no. 11 (2023): EVIDoa2300145, https://doi.org /10.1056/EVIDoa2300145.

Enrique, E., F. Pineda, T. Malek et al., "Sublingual Immunotherapy for Hazelnut Food Allergy: A Randomized, Double-Blind, Placebo-Controlled Study with a Standardized Hazelnut Extract," *Journal of Allergy and Clinical Immunology* 116, no. 5 (2005): 1073–79, https://doi.org/10.1016 /j.jaci.2005.08.027.

Epstein, T. G., K. Murphy-Berendts, G. M. Liss et al., "Risk Factors for Fatal and Nonfatal Reactions to Immunotherapy (2008–2018): Postinjection Monitoring and Severe Asthma," *Annals of Allergy, Asthma & Immunology* 127, no. 1 (2021): 64–69 e1, https://doi.org/10.1016 /j.anai.2021.03.011.

Goldberg, M. R., N. Epstein-Rigbi, A. Elizur, "Eosinophil-Associated Gastrointestinal Manifestations During OIT," *Clinical Reviews in Allergy & Immunology* 65, no. 3 (2023): 365–76, https://doi.org/10.1007/s1 2016-023-08974-0.

Greenhawt, M., J. Oppenheimer, M. Nelson et al., "Sublingual Immunotherapy: A Focused Allergen Immunotherapy Practice Parameter Update," *Annals of Allergy, Asthma & Immunology* 118, no. 3 (2017): 276–82 e2, https://doi.org/10.1016/j.anai.2016.12.009.

Greenhawt, M., S. B. Sindher, J. Wang et al., "Phase 3 Trial of Epicutaneous Immunotherapy in Toddlers with Peanut Allergy," *New England Journal of Medicine* 388, no. 19 (2023): 1755–66, https://doi.org/10.1056/NEJMoa 2212895.

Grzeskowiak, L. E., B. Tao, E. Knight et al., "Adverse Events Associated with Peanut Oral Immunotherapy in Children—A Systematic Review and Meta-Analysis," *Scientific Reports* 10, no. 1 (2020): 659, https://doi.org /10.1038/s41598-019-56961-3.

Hankin, C. S., L. Cox, A. Bronstone et al., "Allergy Immunotherapy: Reduced Health Care Costs in Adults and Children with Allergic Rhinitis," *Journal of Allergy and Clinical Immunology* 131, no. 4 (2013): 1084–91, https://doi .org/10.1016/j.jaci.2012.12.662.

Iliopoulos, O., D. Proud, N. F. Adkinson Jr. et al., "Effects of Immunotherapy on the Early, Late, and Rechallenge Nasal Reaction to Provocation with Allergen: Changes in Inflammatory Mediators and Cells," *Journal of Allergy and Clinical Immunology* 87, no. 4 (1991): 855–66, https://doi .org/10.1016/0091-6749(91)90134-a.

Jakalski, M., A. Bozek, and G. W. Canonica, "Responders and Nonresponders to Pharmacotherapy and Allergen Immunotherapy," *Human Vaccines &*

Immunotherapeutics 15, no. 12 (2019): 2896–902, https://doi.org/10.1080/21645515.2019.1614397.

Jin, H., B. Trogen, and A. Nowak-Wegrzyn, "Eosinophilic Esophagitis as a Complication of Food Oral Immunotherapy," *Current Opinion in Allergy and Clinical Immunology* 20, no. 6 (2020): 616–23, https://doi.org/10.1097/ACI.0000000000000688.

Johnstone, D. E., and A. Dutton, "The Value of Hyposensitization Therapy for Bronchial Asthma in Children—A 14-Year Study," *Pediatrics* 42, no. 5 (1968): 793–802, https://www.ncbi.nlm.nih.gov/pubmed/5685362.

Johnstone, D. E., and L. Crump, "Value of Hyposensitization Therapy for Perennial Bronchial Asthma in Children," *Pediatrics* 27 (1961): 39–44, https://www.ncbi.nlm.nih.gov/pubmed/13790388.

Jones, S. M., S. H. Sicherer, A. W. Burks et al., "Epicutaneous Immunotherapy for the Treatment of Peanut Allergy in Children and Young Adults," *Journal of Allergy and Clinical Immunology* 139, no. 4 (2017): 1242–52 e9, https://doi.org/10.1016/j.jaci.2016.08.017.

Jones, S. M., W. K. Agbotounou, D. M. Fleischer et al., "Safety of Epicutaneous Immunotherapy for the Treatment of Peanut Allergy: A Phase 1 Study Using the Viaskin Patch," *Journal of Allergy and Clinical Immunology* 137, no. 4 (2016): 1258–61 e10, https://doi.org/10.1016/j.jaci.2016.01.008.

Keet, C. A., P. A. Frischmeyer-Guerrerio, A. Thyagarajan et al., "The Safety and Efficacy of Sublingual and Oral Immunotherapy for Milk Allergy," *Journal of Allergy and Clinical Immunology* 129, no. 2 (2012): 448–55 e1–5, https://doi.org/10.1016/j.jaci.2011.10.023.

Kim, E. H., J. A. Bird, M. Kulis et al., "Sublingual Immunotherapy for Peanut Allergy: Clinical and Immunologic Evidence of Desensitization," *Journal of Allergy and Clinical Immunology* 127, no. 3 (2011): 640–46 e1, https://doi.org/10.1016/j.jaci.2010.12.1083.

Kristiansen, M., S. Dhami, G. Netuveli et al., "Allergen Immunotherapy for the Prevention of Allergy: A Systematic Review and Meta-Analysis," *Pediatric Allergy and Immunology* 28, no. 1 (2017): 18–29, https://doi.org/10.1111/pai.12661.

Lamminpaa, I., E. Niccolai, and A. Amedei, "Probiotics as Adjuvants to Mitigate Adverse Reactions and Enhance Effectiveness in Food Allergy Immunotherapy," *Scandinavian Journal of Immunology* 100, no. 6 (2024): e13405, https://doi.org/10.1111/sji.13405.

Lucendo, A. J., A. Arias, and J. M. Tenias, "Relation Between Eosinophilic Esophagitis and Oral Immunotherapy for Food Allergy: A Systematic Review with Meta-Analysis," *Annals of Allergy, Asthma & Immunology* 113, no. 6 (2014): 624–29, https://doi.org/10.1016/j.anai.2014.08.004.

Miehlke, S., O. Alpan, S. Schroder et al., "Induction of Eosinophilic Esophagitis by Sublingual Pollen Immunotherapy," *Case Reports in Gastroenterology* 7, no. 3 (2013): 363–68, https://doi.org/10.1159/000355161.

Nachshon, L., N. Schwartz, M. B. Levy et al., "Severe Anaphylactic Reactions to Home Doses of Oral Immunotherapy for Food Allergy," *Journal of Allergy and Clinical Immunology: In Practice* 11, no. 8 (2023): 2524–33 e3, https://doi.org/10.1016/j.jaip.2023.03.005.

Naclerio, R. M., D. Proud, B. Moylan et al., "A Double-Blind Study of the Discontinuation of Ragweed Immunotherapy," *Journal of Allergy and Clinical Immunology* 100, no. 3 (1997): 293–300, https://doi.org/10.1016/s0091-6749(97)70240-9.

Narisety, S. D., P. A. Frischmeyer-Guerrerio, C. A. Keet et al., "A Randomized, Double-Blind, Placebo-Controlled Pilot Study of Sublingual Versus Oral Immunotherapy for the Treatment of Peanut Allergy," *Journal of Allergy and Clinical Immunology* 135, no. 5 (2015): 1275–82 e1–6, https://doi.org/10.1016/j.jaci.2014.11.005.

Nelson, H. S., M. Makatsori, M. A. Calderon et al., "Subcutaneous Immunotherapy and Sublingual Immunotherapy: Comparative Efficacy, Current and Potential Indications, and Warnings—United States Versus Europe," *Immunology and Allergy Clinics of North America* 36, no. 1 (2016): 13–24, https://doi.org/10.1016/j.iac.2015.08.005.

Passalacqua, G., L. Guerra, E. Compalati et al., "The Safety of Allergen Specific Sublingual Immunotherapy," *Current Drug Safety* 2, no. 2 (2007): 117–23, https://doi.org/10.2174/157488607780598340.

Purello-D'Ambrosio, F., S. Gangemi, R. A. Merendino et al., "Prevention of New Sensitizations in Monosensitized Subjects Submitted to Specific Immunotherapy or Not: A Retrospective Study," *Clinical and Experimental Allergy* 31, no. 8 (2001):1295–302, https://doi.org/10.1046/j.1365-2222.2001.01027.x

Tang, M. L., A. L. Ponsonby, F. Orsini et al., "Administration of a Probiotic with Peanut Oral Immunotherapy: A Randomized Trial," *Journal of Allergy and Clinical Immunology* 135, no. 3 (2015): 737–44 e8, https://doi.org/10.1016/j.jaci.2014.11.034.

Vickery, B. P., and A. W. Burks, "Immunotherapy in the Treatment of Food Allergy: Focus on Oral Tolerance," *Current Opinion in Allergy and Clinical Immunology* 9, no. 4 (2009): 364–70, https://doi.org/10.1097 /ACI.0b013e32832d9add.

Wang, N., J. Song, S. R. Sun et al., "Immune Signatures Predict Response to House Dust Mite Subcutaneous Immunotherapy in Patients with Allergic Rhinitis," *Allergy: European Journal of Allergy and Clinical Immunology* 79, no. 5 (2024): 1230–41, https://doi.org/10.1111/all.16068.

You, L. C., G. Soffer, and J. Factor, "Clinical Experience with Sesame Oral Immunotherapy and a Quality-of-Life Assessment," *Journal of Food Allergy* 4, no. 1 (2022):1–9, https://doi.org/10.2500/jfa.2022.4.220003.

Chapter 17—Biologics

Blauvelt, A., M. de Bruin-Weller, M. Gooderham et al., "Long-Term Management of Moderate-to-Severe Atopic Dermatitis with Dupilumab and Concomitant Topical Corticosteroids (Liberty Ad Chronos): A 1-Year, Randomised, Double-Blinded, Placebo-Controlled, Phase 3 Trial," *The Lancet* 389, no. 10086 (2017): 2287–303, https://doi.org/10.1016 /S0140-6736(17)31191-1.

Busse, W., R. Buhl, C. Fernandez Vidaurre et al., "Omalizumab and the Risk of Malignancy: Results from a Pooled Analysis," *Journal of Allergy and Clinical Immunology* 129, no. 4 (2012): 983–89 e6, https://doi.org /10.1016/j.jaci.2012.01.033.

Chehade, M., E. S. Dellon, J. M. Spergel et al., "Dupilumab for Eosinophilic Esophagitis in Patients 1 to 11 Years of Age," *New England Journal of Medicine* 390, no. 24 (2024): 2239–51, https://doi.org/10.1056 /NEJMoa2312282.

Corren, J., T. B. Casale, B. Lanier et al., "Safety and Tolerability of Omalizumab," *Clinical and Experimental Allergy* 39, no. 6 (2009): 788–97, https://doi.org/10.1111/j.1365-2222.2009.03214.x.

Cox, L., P. Lieberman, D. Wallace et al., "American Academy of Allergy, Asthma & Immunology/American College of Allergy, Asthma & Immunology Omalizumab-Associated Anaphylaxis Joint Task Force Follow-up Report," *Journal of Allergy and Clinical Immunology* 128, no. 1 (2011): 210–12, https://doi.org/10.1016/j.jaci.2011.04.010.

Cox, L., T. A. E. Platts-Mills, I. Finegold et al., "American Academy of Allergy, Asthma & Immunology/American College of Allergy, Asthma and Immunology Joint Task Force Report on Omalizumab-Associated

Anaphylaxis," *Journal of Allergy and Clinical Immunology* 120, no. 6 (2007): 1373–77, https://doi.org/10.1016/j.jaci.2007.09.032.

Dellon, E. S., M. E. Rothenberg, M. H. Collins et al., "Dupilumab in Adults and Adolescents with Eosinophilic Esophagitis," *New England Journal of Medicine* 387, no. 25 (2022): 2317–30, https://doi.org/10.1056/NEJMoa2205982.

Deniz, Y. M., and N. Gupta, "Safety and Tolerability of Omalizumab (Xolair), a Recombinant Humanized Monoclonal Anti-IgE Antibody," *Clinical Reviews in Allergy & Immunology* 29, no. 1 (2005): 31–48, https://doi.org/10.1385/criai:29:1:031.

Fachler, T., R. Shreberk-Hassidim, and V. Molho-Pessach, "Dupilumab-Induced Ocular Surface Disease: A Systematic Review," *Journal of the American Academy of Dermatology* 86, no. 2 (2022): 486–87, https://doi.org/10.1016/j.jaad.2021.09.029.

Fokkens, W. J., A. S. Viskens, V. Backer et al., "Epos/Euforea Update on Indication and Evaluation of Biologics in Chronic Rhinosinusitis with Nasal Polyps 2023," *Rhinology* 61, no. 3 (2023): 194–202, https://doi.org/10.4193/Rhin22.489.

Furue, K., T. Ito, G. Tsuji et al., "The IL-13-OVOL1-FLG Axis in Atopic Dermatitis," *Immunology* 158, no. 4 (2019): 281–86, https://doi.org/10.1111/imm.13120.

Hernandez, I., S. W. Bott, A. S. Patel et al., "Pricing of Monoclonal Antibody Therapies: Higher If Used for Cancer?" *American Journal of Managed Care* 24, no. 2 (2018): 109–12, https://www.ncbi.nlm.nih.gov/pubmed/29461857.

Hirano, I., E. S. Dellon, J. D. Hamilton, et al., "Efficacy of Dupilumab in a Phase 2 Randomized Trial of Adults with Active Eosinophilic Esophagitis," *Gastroenterology* 158, no. 1 (2020): 111–22 e10, https://doi.org/10.1053/j.gastro.2019.09.042.

Long, A., A. Rahmaoui, K. J. Rothman et al., "Incidence of Malignancy in Patients with Moderate-to-Severe Asthma Treated with or Without Omalizumab," *Journal of Allergy and Clinical Immunology* 134, no. 3 (2014): 560–67 e4, https://doi.org/10.1016/j.jaci.2014.02.007.

Napolitano, M., F. di Vico, A. Ruggiero et al., "The Hidden Sentinel of the Skin: An Overview on the Role of Interleukin-13 in Atopic Dermatitis," *Frontiers in Medicine (Lausanne)* 10 (2023): 1165098, https://doi.org/10.3389/fmed.2023.1165098.

Paller, A. S., E. L. Simpson, E. C. Siegfried et al., "Dupilumab in Children Aged 6 Months to Younger Than 6 Years with Uncontrolled Atopic Dermatitis: A Randomised, Double-Blind, Placebo-Controlled, Phase 3 Trial," *The Lancet* 400, no. 10356 (2022): 908–19, https://doi.org/10.1016/S0140-6736(22)01539-2.

Simpson, E. L., T. Bieber, E. Guttman-Yassky et al., "Two Phase 3 Trials of Dupilumab Versus Placebo in Atopic Dermatitis," *New England Journal of Medicine* 375, no. 24 (2016): 2335–48, https://doi.org/10.1056/NEJMoa1610020.

Soria, A., A. Du-Thanh, J. Seneschal et al., "Development or Exacerbation of Head and Neck Dermatitis in Patients Treated for Atopic Dermatitis with Dupilumab," *JAMA Dermatology* 155, no. 11 (2019): 1312–15, https://doi.org/10.1001/jamadermatol.2019.2613.

Wood, R. A., A. Togias, S. H. Sicherer et al., "Omalizumab for the Treatment of Multiple Food Allergies," *New England Journal of Medicine* 390, no. 10 (2024): 889–99, https://doi.org/10.1056/NEJMoa2312382.

Wu, A. C., A. L. Fuhlbrigge, M. A. Robayo et al., "Cost-Effectiveness of Biologics for Allergic Diseases," *Journal of Allergy and Clinical Immunology: Practice* 9, no. 3 (2021): 1107–17 e2, https://doi.org/10.1016/j.jaip.2020.10.009.

Zhao, Z. T., C. M. Ji, W. J. Yu et al., "Omalizumab for the Treatment of Chronic Spontaneous Urticaria: A Meta-Analysis of Randomized Clinical Trials," *Journal of Allergy and Clinical Immunology* 137, no. 6 (2016): 1742–50 e4, https://doi.org/10.1016/j.jaci.2015.12.1342.

Chapter 18—Future Directions

"Allergy Amulet," Allergy Amulet, accessed December 15, 2024, https://www.allergyamulet.com.

"Aquestive Therapeutics Provides Business Update and Outlines Key 2025 Objectives," Aquestive Therapeutics, accessed January 13, 2025, https://investors.aquestive.com/news-releases/news-release-details/aquestive-therapeutics-provides-business-update-and-outlines-0.

"Intellia Therapeutics Announces First Patient Dosed in the HAELO Phase 3 Study of NTLA-2002, an Investigational in Vivo CRISPR Gene Editing Treatment for Hereditary Angioedema," Intellia Therapeutics, January 22, 2025, https://ir.intelliatx.com/news-releases/news-release-details/intellia-therapeutics-announces-first-patient-dosed-haelo-phase.

"Novartis Phase III Data Confirm Sustained Efficacy and Long-Term Safety of Oral Remibrutinib in Chronic Spontaneous Urticaria," Novartis, May 31, 2024, accessed January 4, 2025, https://www.novartis.com/news/media-releases/novartis-phase-iii-data-confirm-sustained-efficacy-and-long-term-safety-oral-remibrutinib-chronic-spontaneous-urticaria.

"Short-Term Linvoseltamab Treatment on Top of Chronic Dupilumab Treatment for Adults with Severe Immunoglobulin E (IgE)-Mediated Food Allergy," National Library of Medicine, accessed January 8, 2025, https://clinicaltrials.gov/study/NCT06369467.

Abdelhalim, A., O. Yilmaz, M. Elshaikh Berai et al., "A Narrative Review of the OX40-OX40L Pathway as a Potential Therapeutic Target in Atopic Dermatitis: Focus on Rocatinlimab and Amlitelimab," *Dermatology and Therapy (Heidelberg)* 14, no. 12 (2024): 3197–210, https://doi.org/10.1007/s13555-024-01308-8.

Berger, W. E., N. Faris, M. Weinstein et al., "Randomized, Placebo-Controlled, Phase 1 Safety Study of Oral Mucosal Immunotherapy in Adults with Peanut Allergy," *Annals of Allergy, Asthma & Immunology* 134, no. 4 (2025), 448–56, https://doi.org/10.1016/j.anai.2025.01.013.

Boyd, H., and A. F. Santos, "Novel Diagnostics in Food Allergy," *Journal of Allergy and Clinical Immunology* 155, no. 2 (2024): 275–85, https://doi.org/10.1016/j.jaci.2024.12.1071.

Calazans, A. P. C. T., T. M. S. Milani, A. S. Prata et al., "A Functional Bread Fermented with *Saccharomyces cerevisiae* UFMG A-905 Prevents Allergic Asthma in Mice," *Current Developments in Nutrition* 8, no. 4 (2024): 102142, https://doi.org/10.1016/j.cdnut.2024.102142.

Craig, T. J., A. Reshef, H. H. Li et al., "Efficacy and Safety of Garadacimab, a Factor XIIa Inhibitor for Hereditary Angioedema Prevention (Vanguard): A Global, Multicenter, Randomized, Double-Blind, Placebo-Controlled, Phase 3 Trial," *The Lancet* 401, no. 10382 (2023): 1079–90, https://doi.org/10.1016/S0140-6736(23)00350-1.

Du, F., C. H. Rische, Y. Li et al., "Controlled Adsorption of Multiple Bioactive Proteins Enables Targeted Mast Cell Nanotherapy," *Nature Nanotechnology* 19, no. 5 (2024): 698–704, https://doi.org/10.1038/s41565-023-01584-z.

Eggel, A., L. F. Pennington, and T. S. Jardetzky, "Therapeutic Monoclonal Antibodies in Allergy: Targeting IgE, Cytokine, and Alarmin Pathways," *Immunological Reviews* 328, no. 1 (2024): 387–411, https://doi.org/10.1111/imr.13380.

Evans, E. L., K. Cuthbertson, N. Endesh et al., "Yoda1 Analogue (Dooku1) Which Antagonizes Yoda1-Evoked Activation of Piezo1 and Aortic Relaxation," *British Journal of Pharmacology* 175, no. 10 (2018):1744–59, https://doi.org/10.1111/bph.14188.

Goldberg, M. R., M. Y. Appel, K. Tobi et al., "Validation of the NUT CRACKER Diagnostic Algorithm and Prediction for Cashew and Pistachio Co-Allergy," *Journal of Allergy and Clinical Immunology: In Practice* 12, no. 5 (2024): 1273–82, https://doi.org/10.1016/j.jaip.2024.02.012.

Hurrell, B. P., S. Shen, X. Li et al., "Piezo1 Channels Restrain ILC2s and Regulate the Development of Airway Hyperreactivity," *Journal of Experimental Medicine* 221, no. 5 (2024): e29231835, https://doi.org/10.1084/jem.20231835.

Hwang, D. W., C. R. Nagler, and C. E. Ciaccio, "New and Emerging Concepts and Therapies for the Treatment of Food Allergy," *Immunotherapy Advances* 2, no. 1 (2022): ltac006, https://doi.org/10.1093/immadv/ltac006.

Jackson, D. J., M. E. Wechsler, D. J. Jackson et al., "Twice-Yearly Depemokimab in Severe Asthma with an Eosinophilic Phenotype," *New England Journal of Medicine* 391, no. 24 (2024): 2337–49, https://doi.org/10.1056/NEJMoa2406673.

Maniu, A. A., M. I. Perde-Schrepler, C. B. Tatomi et al., "Latest Advances in Chronic Rhinosinusitis with Nasal Polyps Endotyping and Biomarkers, and Their Significance for Daily Practice," *Romanian Journal of Morphology and Embryology* 61, no. 2 (2020): 309–20, https://doi.org/10.47162/RJME.61.2.01.

Martin, S. F., T. Rustemeyer, and J. P. Thyssen, "Recent Advances in Understanding and Managing Contact Dermatitis," *F1000Research* 7 (2018): 810, https://doi.org/10.12688/f1000research.13499.1.

Patel, G. B., R. C. Kern, J. A. Bernstein et al., "Current and Future Treatments of Rhinitis and Sinusitis," *Journal of Allergy and Clinical Immunology: In Practice* 8, no. 5 (2020): 1522–31, https://doi.org/10.1016/j.jaip.2020.01.031.

Pfaar, O., J. Portnoy, H. Nolte et al., "Future Directions of Allergen Immunotherapy for Allergic Rhinitis: Experts' Perspective," *Journal of Allergy and Clinical Immunology: In Practice* 12, no. 1 (2024): 32–44, https://doi.org/10.1016/j.jaip.2023.08.047.

Phipatanakul, W., D. T. Mauger, T. W. Guilbert et al., "Preventing Asthma in High-Risk Kids (PARK) with Omalizumab: Design, Rationale, Methods,

Lessons Learned and Adaptation," *Contemporary Clinical Trials* 100 (2021): 106228, https://doi.org/10.1016/j.cct.2020.106228.

Powell, N., M. Blank, A. Luintel et al., "Narrative Review of Recent Developments and the Future of Penicillin Allergy De-Labelling by Non-Allergists," *NPJ Antimicrobials and Resistance* 2, no. 1 (2024): 18, https://doi.org/10.1038/s44259-024-00035-6.

Ramakrishnan, S., R. E. K. Russell, H. R. Mahmoo et al., "Treating Eosinophilic Exacerbations of Asthma and COPD with Benralizumab (ABRA): A Double-Blind, Double-Dummy, Active Placebo-Controlled Randomised Trial," *Lancet Respiratory Medicine* 13, no. 1 (2025): 59–68, https://doi.org/10.1016/S2213-2600(24)00299-6.

Sabato, V., M. Beyens, A. Toscano et al., "Mast Cell-Targeting Therapies in Mast Cell Activation Syndromes," *Current Allergy and Asthma Reports* 24, no. 2 (2024): 63–71, https://doi.org/10.1007/s11882-023-01123-9.

Santos, A. F., G. Du Toit, C. O'Rourke et al., "Biomarkers of Severity and Threshold of Allergic Reactions During Oral Peanut Challenges," *Journal of Allergy and Clinical Immunology* 146, no. 2 (2020): 344–55, https://doi .org/10.1016/j.jaci.2020.03.035.

Sideris, N., E. Paschou, K. Bakirtzi et al., "New and Upcoming Topical Treatments for Atopic Dermatitis: A Review of the Literature," *Journal of Clinical Medicine* 11, no. 17 (2022), https://doi.org/10.3390 /jcm11174974.

Sobczak, J. M., P. S. Krenger, F. Storni et al., "The Next Generation Virus-Like Particle Platform for the Treatment of Peanut Allergy," *Allergy: European Journal of Allergy and Clinical Immunology* 78, no. 7 (2023): 1980–86, https://doi.org/10.1111/all.15704.

Sundhoro, M., S. R. Agnihotra, N. D. Khan et al., "Rapid and Accurate Electrochemical Sensor for Food Allergen Detection in Complex Foods," *Scientific Reports* 11, no. 1 (2021): 20831, https://doi.org/10 .1038/s41598-021-00241-6.

Ten Have, P., P. van Hal, I. Wichers et al., "Turning Green: The Impact of Changing to More Eco-Friendly Respiratory Healthcare—A Carbon and Cost Analysis of Dutch Prescription Data," *BMJ Open* 12, no. 6 (2022): e055546, https://doi.org/10.1136/bmjopen-2021-055546.

Voskamp, A. L., S. Khosa, T. Phan et al., "Phase 1 Trial Supports Safety and Mechanism of Action of Peptide Immunotherapy for Peanut Allergy," *Allergy* 79, no. 2 (2024): 485–98, https://doi.org/10.1111 /all.15966.

Wijerathne, T. D., A. D. Ozkan, and J. J. Lacroix, "Yoda1's Energetic Footprint on Piezo1 Channels and Its Modulation by Voltage and Temperature," *Proceedings of the National Academy of Sciences of the United States of America* 119, no. 29 (2022): e2202269119, https://doi.org/10.1073/pnas.2202269119.

Xu, X., X. Wang, Y. P. Liao et al., "Use of a Liver-Targeting Immune-Tolerogenic mRNA Lipid Nanoparticle Platform to Treat Peanut-Induced Anaphylaxis by Single- and Multiple-Epitope Nucleotide Sequence Delivery," *ACS Nano* 17, no. 5 (2023): 4942–57, https://doi.org/10.1021/acsnano.2c12420.

Zhang, Y., F. Lan, and L. Zhang, "Advances and Highlights in Allergic Rhinitis," *Allergy: European Journal of Allergy and Clinical Immunology* 76, no. 11 (2021): 3383–89, https://doi.org/10.1111/all.15044.

Zuberbier, T., L. F. Ensina, A. Gimenez-Arnau et al., "Chronic Urticaria: Unmet Needs, Emerging Drugs, and New Perspectives on Personalised Treatment," *The Lancet* 404, no. 10450 (2024): 393–404, https://doi.org/10.1016/S0140-6736(24)00852-3.

Index

Note: Italicized page numbers indicate material in photographs or illustrations.

About the Author

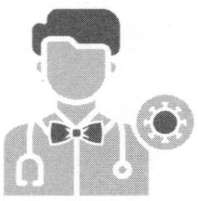

Zachary Rubin, MD, is a double board-certified physician in pediatrics and allergy/immunology, who is passionate about helping individuals of all ages breathe easier, live symptom-free, and take control of their allergic conditions. He currently practices at Oak Brook Allergists in the Chicago area.

Nationally recognized for his approachable style and clear explanations, Dr. Rubin is also a prominent medical educator and public health advocate with over four million followers across social media. Through his platforms under the handle @Rubin_Allergy, he translates complex science into understandable and actionable advice, tackling everything from environmental allergies to the latest vaccine news—often with a dash of humor and the occasional bow tie.

Dr. Rubin earned his medical degree at Case Western Reserve University School of Medicine and went on to complete a pediatrics residency at the University of Illinois College of Medicine in Chicago and an allergy/immunology fellowship at Washington University School of Medicine in St. Louis. He is an outspoken advocate for evidence-based medicine, accessible treatment, and combating health misinformation.

When he's not seeing patients or creating educational content, Dr. Rubin enjoys swimming, hiking, Hula-Hooping, spending time with his wife, Melanie, and daughter, Juliana, and going on adventures with their three beloved German shepherds—Leia, Sadie, and Tucker.

All About Allergies is his first book.